Fetal Medicine for the MRCOG and Beyond

Second edition

Fetal Medicine for the MRCOG and Beyond

WITHDRAWN

Second edition

Alan Cameron MD FRCOG
Consultant in Fetal and Maternal Medicine
The Southern General Hospital, Glasgow, UK

Janet Brennand MD FRCOG
Consultant in Fetal and Maternal Medicine
The Southern General Hospital, Glasgow, UK

Lena Crichton MD FRCOG
Consultant Obstetrician
Royal Aberdeen Maternity Hospital, Aberdeen, UK

Janice Gibson MD MRCOG
Consultant in Fetal and Maternal Medicine
The Southern General Hospital, Glasgow, UK

Series Editor: **Jenny Higham**

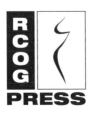

ISBN 978-1-906985-36-3

A machine-readable catalogue record for this publication can be obtained from the British Library [www.bl.uk/catalogues/listings.html]

Published by the **RCOG Press** at the
Royal College of Obstetricians and Gynaecologists
27 Sussex Place, Regent's Park
London NW1 4RG

Registered Charity No. 213280

Cover image:
A longitudinal section through the fetus demonstrating a normal facial profile

RCOG Press Editor: Jane Moody
Index: Liza Furnival
Design & typesetting: Tony Crowley
Printed in the UK by Latimer Trend & Co. Ltd, Estover Road, Plymouth PL6 7PL

Contents

Preface

It is essential for both those hoping to specialise in obstetrics and gynae-cology and established practitioners to have a solid understanding of fetal medicine to help answer the question foremost in every prospective parent's mind: 'Is my baby going to be normal?' This comprehensive book, written by undisputed experts in fetal medicine, covers the whole field, addressing screening methods, diagnostic techniques and the manage-ment of fetal abnormality following diagnosis.

This second edition has been extensively updated to reflect current clinical practice and developments in the field since the publication of the original edition, and incorporates a thoroughly revised structure and contents. It will be of great assistance not only to MRCOG candidates in their preparation for the examination but also to any health professional who comes into contact with mothers and babies, including midwives, and who wants to update their knowledge. I hope you find this latest book in the MRCOG and Beyond series helpful.

Professor Jenny Higham
Series Editor

Abbreviations

AFP	alphafetoprotein
AIDS	autoimmune disease syndrome
CAH	congenital adrenal hyperplasia
CCAM	congenital cystadenomatoid malformation
CDH	congenital diaphragmatic hernia
CEMAT	Canadian Early and Mid-trimester Amniocentesis Trial
CHD	congenital heart disease
CI	confidence interval
CMV	cytomegalovirus
CRL	crown–rump length
CTG	cardiotocogram
CVR	cystic adenomatoid volume ratio
CVS	chorionic villus sampling
D&E	dilatation and evacuation
ELISA	enzyme-linked immunosorbent assay
FaSTER	First- and Second-Trimester Evaluation of Risk for aneuploidy
FETO	Fetal Endoscopic Tracheal Occlusion (Task Force)
FISH	fluorescence *in situ* hybridisation
FNAIT	fetal and neonatal alloimmune thrombocytopenia
FTA-abs	fluorescent treponemal antibody-absorbed
FVS	fetal varicella syndrome
FVW	flow velocity waveform
HAART	highly-active antiretroviral therapy
hCG	human chorionic gonadotrophin
HIV	human immunodeficiency syndrome
HLHS	hypoplastic left heart syndrome
HPA	human platelet antigens
IgE	immunoglobulin E
IgG	immunoglobulin G
IgM	immunoglobulin M
LUTO	lower urinary tract obstruction
MCA	middle cerebral artery

MoM	multiples of the median
Nd:YAG	neodymium: yttrium-aluminium-garnet
NHS FASP	National Health Service Fetal Anomaly Screening Programme
NIHF	non-immune hydrops fetalis
NSAIDS	non-steroidal anti-inflammatory drugs
OR	odds ratio
PAPP-A	pregnancy-associated plasma protein A
PCR	polymerase chain reaction
PI	pulsatility index
PlGF	placental growth factor
PPROM	preterm prelabour rupture of the membranes
PSV	peak systolic velocity
QFPCR	quantitative fluorescence polymerase chain reaction
RPR	rapid plasma regain
SGA	small for gestational age
SURUSS	Serum Urine and Ultrasound Screening Study
SVT	supraventricular tachycardia
TPHA	Treponema pallidum haemagglutination test
TRAP	twin reversed arterial perfusion
TTTS	twin–twin transfusion syndrome
uE_3	unconjugated estriol
VDRL	Venereal Diseases Research Laboratory
VEGF	vascular endothelial growth factor
VSD	ventricular septal defect
VZ IgG	varicella zoster immunoglobulin G
VZV	varicella zoster virus

1 Screening for chromosomal abnormalities

Introduction

Screening for chromosomal abnormalities in an obstetric setting has traditionally meant screening for trisomy 21 (Down syndrome). Down syndrome has a livebirth incidence of approximately one in 700 and is the single most common cause of mental restriction in school-age children. It is associated with a spectrum of mental and physical handicap and, in view of this, strategies have been developed to identify those pregnancies at 'high risk' of the condition. This affords the opportunity for subsequent diagnostic testing and termination of an affected pregnancy, if chosen by the parents. Screening for trisomy 21 is offered routinely as part of antenatal care and forms the major focus of discussion for this chapter.

The success of a screening programme is not measured only by the number of affected pregnancies detected. Screening for trisomy 21 should be performed on an 'opt-in' basis and it is essential that parents who choose to enter a screening programme have adequate information about the implications and limitations of the test, so that they are not faced with results and decisions for which they are unprepared. Appropriate counselling is therefore paramount to ensure that parents for whom screening is inappropriate do not enter the programme.

A screening test simply places the individual in a 'high-risk' or a 'low-risk' group. It does not tell us whether or not the condition being screened for is actually present. Thus, a woman who has a 'high-risk' screening test result for trisomy 21 would have to undergo a diagnostic test if she wished to establish whether or not the pregnancy was affected. Similarly, a 'low-risk' result does not exclude the presence of trisomy 21; there is no such thing as 'no-risk' on the basis of a screening test result.

Development of screening programmes

Screening programmes have advanced from a single marker – maternal age – to using a combination of markers, including biochemical and ultrasound features. In addition, there has been a drive to offer screening at

Table 1.1 Description of individual screening strategies (Adapted from Wald et al.)[18]

Screening strategy	Description
Nuchal translucency (NT)	First-trimester test based on NT measurement and maternal age
Combined test	First-trimester test combining NT measurement, maternal age, PAPP-A and free βhCG
Double test	Second-trimester test measuring AFP and hCG (either free βhCG or total), together with maternal age
Triple test	Second-trimester test measuring AFP, uE$_3$ and hCG (either free βhCG or total), together with maternal age
Quadruple test	Second-trimester test measuring AFP, uE$_3$ and hCG (either free βhCG or total) and inhibin A, together with maternal age
Integrated test	Integration of first-trimester nuchal translucency and PAPP-A with the second-trimester quadruple test
Serum Integrated test	Integration of first-trimester PAPP-A with second-trimester quadruple test (no NT measurements)
Sequential test	A first-trimester test is performed; women at high risk are offered immediate diagnostic testing. All remaining women proceed to second-trimester serum markers, which are combined with the first-trimester markers to form an integrated test
Contingent screening	A first-trimester test is performed; women found to be high-risk screen positive are offered immediate diagnostic testing. Women who are screen negative receive no further testing. An intermediate group (lower-risk screen positive) proceed to second-trimester quadruple testing to form an integrated test in combination with the first-trimester markers

AFP = alphafetoprotein; hCG = human chorionic gonadotrophin; PAPP-A = pregnancy-associated plasma protein A; uE$_3$ = unconjugated estriol

earlier gestations. The development of new screening programmes will be discussed in turn. The various programmes are summarised in Table 1.1.

Maternal age

Ninety-five percent of cases of trisomy 21 are due to non-disjunction, an abnormality of meiotic division, and the risk is known to increase with advancing maternal age. The risk of trisomy 21 increases relatively gradu-

Table 1.2 The frequency of trisomy 21 at birty and at mid-trimester (time of amniocentesis) according to maternal age (Connor and Ferguson-Smith 1997)[31]

Maternal age	Frequency at birth	Frequency mid-trimester
20	1 in 1500	1 in 1200
25	1 in 1350	1 in 1000
30	1 in 900	1 in 700
35	1 in 380	1 in 300
37	1 in 240	1 in 200
39	1 in 150	1 in 120
41	1 in 85	1 in 70
45	1 in 28	1 in 22

ally up until the age of 35 years, after which time the increase in risk is much steeper (Table 1.2). The first screening programme for trisomy 21 was therefore based on maternal age, since it was estimated that approximately 30% of trisomy 21 pregnancies occurred to mothers of 35 years and above. However, since not all women in this age group opted for diagnostic testing (amniocentesis), actual detection rates were much lower than the potential 30%.

Biochemical screening

SECOND-TRIMESTER BIOCHEMICAL SCREENING

Alphafetoprotein (AFP) was the first serum marker to be used in screening programmes for trisomy 21. AFP is a fetal-specific protein that is produced initially by the fetal yolk sac and subsequently by the fetal liver. Biochemical screening has traditionally been performed between 15 and 21 weeks of gestation, during which time maternal serum levels of AFP increase secondary to transport across the placenta and amnion. In pregnancies affected by trisomy 21, AFP levels are reduced compared with unaffected pregnancies and maternal serum AFP in combination with age increased detection rates to approximately 40%.

In screening programmes, marker levels are described in multiples of the median (MoM) to allow for the fact that levels vary with gestational age. Values are calculated by dividing an individual's marker level by the median level of that marker for the relevant gestation. The use of MoM values allows results from different laboratories to be interpreted in a

Table 1.3	Second-trimester serum markers, median multiples of the median (MOM) in pregnancies affected by trisomy 21 (reproduced with permission from Wald et al.)[1]
Marker	MOM in trisomy 21
Alphafetoprotein	0.75
Human chorionic gonadotrophin (hCG)	2.06
Free βhCG	2.20
Unconjugated estriol	0.72
Inhibin A	1.92

common manner and facilitates adjustments for variables that influence marker levels. The performance of a particular screening test is defined by its detection rate for a given false positive rate, the latter being the percentage of unaffected pregnancies categorised as 'high risk' by the screening test and thus potentially subject to diagnostic testing.

A number of other serum markers are of value in second-trimester screening for trisomy 21. These are intact human chorionic gonadotrophin (hCG) or its free β-subunit (free βhCG), unconjugated estriol (uE_3) and inhibin A. Table 1.3 illustrates the effect of trisomy 21 on serum marker levels.[1] Biochemical screening programmes now use maternal age and a combination of markers. The 'double test' combines age with AFP and hCG and has detection rates of approximately 66% for a 5% false positive rate.[2] The 'triple test' adds uE_3 to this combination. Opinion varies about the role of uE_3 in screening, ranging from no additional benefit to an increase in sensitivity of up to 10%.[1,3] Data from the SURUSS[2] and FaSTER[4] trials, described later, demonstrate detection rates of 74% and 70%, respectively, for triple-marker screening, for a 5% false-positive rate. In both of these trials, the addition of inhibin A (quadruple-marker screening) gave a detection rate of 81%, for a 5% false-positive rate.

Factors affecting second-trimester screening

Ultrasound assessment of gestational age results in improved performance of serum markers compared with gestation based on menstrual history. A number of variables influence marker levels (Table 1.4). Adjustments are routinely made for maternal weight in screening programmes. Serum marker levels are higher in twin pregnancies (see later text). Women who have had a screen-positive result in a previous pregnancy are more likely to have screen- positive result in subsequent pregnancies. The chance of

Table 1.4   Variables affecting biochemical screening serum markers

Variable	Serum marker
Maternal weight	AFP and hCG inversely proportional to weight
Insulin-dependent diabetes	uE_3 inhibin A reduced Total/free βhCG unchanged AFP ?significant effect
Afro-Caribbean race	AFP, hCG increased
Smoking	Total and free βhCG reduced AFP increased

AFP = alphafetoprotein; βhCG = beta human chorionic gonadotrophin; uE_3 = unconjugated estradiol

a recurrent false-positive result in a subsequent pregnancy can be 20%. The reason for this is that there is an association between marker levels in successive pregnancies. It is recognised that women who have experienced a false-positive result in a previous pregnancy are more reluctant to undergo screening in their next pregnancy. This can be overcome by adjusting the serum markers of all women who have been screened in a previous pregnancy and not had a pregnancy affected by trisomy 21. The adjustment is made by dividing the observed MoM for a given marker by the previous pregnancy MoM for that marker. By using the adjusted MoM the false positive rate of a variety of screening programmes can be reduced by about two-thirds for women with a previous false-positive result.[6]

FIRST-TRIMESTER BIOCHEMICAL SCREENING

The role of biochemical markers for screening in the first trimester has been evaluated. All of the markers that have been considered for use in the second trimester have been investigated but only free βhCG and pregnancy-associated plasma protein A (PAPP-A) are clearly discriminatory. In contrast to the second trimester, intact hCG is of no value in first-trimester screening. In pregnancies affected by trisomy 21, free βhCG levels are increased (1.83 MoM) and PAPP-A levels are reduced (0.38 MoM) compared with unaffected pregnancies. After 13 weeks of gestation, PAPP-A loses its discrimination as a screening marker. First-trimester serum screening programmes combining maternal age, free βhCG and PAPP-A, with detection rates of 60–68% have been reported, using a risk cut-off level of 1:250, for a false-positive rate of approximately 5%.[7,8]

NUCHAL TRANSLUCENCY

Nuchal translucency is the description given to the ultrasonic appearance of the fluid-filled space between the fetal skin and the soft tissue overlying the cervical spine (Figure 1.1). It is measured between 10 and 14 weeks of gestation, optimally between 11 and 13 weeks. Prerequisites for nuchal translucency measurement are:[9]

- crown-rump length (CRL) 38–84 mm
- good sagittal view
- fetus occupies 75% or more of the image, neutral position
- ultrasound machine has 0.1-mm calipers
- maximum thickness of the subcutaneous translucency between the skin and soft tissue overlying the cervical spine is measured
- distinguish between fetal skin and amnion.

A number of studies have confirmed that an increased nuchal translucency is associated with aneuploidy. In the first trimester of normal pregnancy, nuchal translucency thickness increases with advancing gestation. The 95th centile for nuchal translucency thickness is 0.8 mm above the normal median throughout the gestational range of 10–14 weeks. It is therefore the difference between the nuchal translucency measurement and the appropriate normal median for gestation that is incorporated into the model to calculate trisomy 21 risk. A large multi-centre study of an unselected population has demonstrated that nuchal translucency measurement in combination with maternal age will identify a 'high-risk' group in which 77% of cases of trisomy 21 are

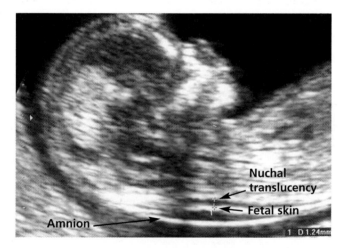

Figure 1.1 Nuchal translucency measurement, indicated by the calipers; fetal skin and amnion are differentiated

detected for a 5% false-positive rate.[9]

Potential problems with nuchal translucency screening for trisomy 21 have been identified. It may be difficult to obtain a measurement if the fetal position is incorrect or there is maternal adiposity, in which case the scan will have to be prolonged or repeated. The effect of this on the management of ultrasound departments and antenatal clinics needs to be considered when introducing such a programme. Concerns have also been raised regarding the reproducibility of the measurement, highlighting the need for training and audit to ensure that the quality of screening programmes is equivalent between centres.

INCREASED NUCHAL TRANSLUCENCY AND NORMAL KARYOTYPE

Increased nuchal translucency is not only associated with aneuploidy. It can indicate a number of fetal complications, including congenital defects and adverse pregnancy outcome. Increased nuchal translucency is associated with congenital diaphragmatic hernia and skeletal dysplasias but cardiac anomalies are the most common congenital defects. The prevalence of cardiac defects increases with thickness of the nuchal translucency (for example, 18.2/1000 for a nuchal translucency between the 95th and 99th centiles and 126.7/1000 for a nuchal translucency greater than 5.5mm).[10] The risk of congenital anomaly, fetal or neonatal death also increases from 5% (nuchal translucency 95th centile 3.4 mm) to 80% for nuchal translucency greater than 5.5 mm.[11]

First-trimester combined ultrasound and biochemical screening

The combination of first-trimester nuchal translucency measurement and biochemical markers for detection of trisomy 21 has been the subject of

Table 1.5 Sensitivity of first-trimester screening programmes, for a 5% false positive rate

Screening programme	Sensitivity (%)
Maternal age + free βhCG	38
Age + PAPP-A	52
Age + PAPP-A + free βhCG	60
Age + nuchal translucency	77
Age + nuchal translucency + PAPP-A + free βhCG	89

βhCG = beta human chorionic gonadotrophin; PAPP-A = pregnancy-associated plasma protein A

much research. In several studies, free βhCG, PAPP-A, nuchal translucency and maternal age in combination has been described, with reported sensitivities of 80–89% for detection of trisomy 21.[12,13] These are substantially higher detection rates than second-trimester biochemical screening, for the same false-positive rate. It has been calculated that the detection rate of a first-trimester programme should be 8.3% higher if it is to be considered superior to second-trimester screening[14] and the addition of nuchal translucency to first-trimester biochemistry clearly meets this criterion. First-trimester screening strategies are summarised in Table 1.5.

INTEGRATED SCREENING

Integrated screening is described in the SURUSS study, which prospectively enrolled 47 053 singleton pregnancies between 1995 and 2002.[2] It provides data on women seen in both the first and second trimesters of pregnancy, without any intervention taking place in the first trimester. There were 101 Down syndrome pregnancies in the study. Women had first trimester (9–13 completed weeks) nuchal translucency measurements and collection of blood and urine samples. In the second trimester (14–22 weeks) blood and urine samples were repeated. Serum samples were assayed for PAPP-A, free βhCG, total hCG, uE_3 and dimeric inhibin A. Urine was assayed for invasive trophoblast antigen, β-core fragment, total hCG and free βhCG. Results were disclosed in the second trimester.

The integrated test had the best screening performance if the first trimester nuchal translucency and PAPP-A were performed at 10 completed weeks of gestation, followed by the quadruple test at 14–22 weeks. In practice, 11 weeks is probably the gestation of choice for obtaining nuchal translucency measurements, hence the results of the SURUSS

Table 1.6	False positive rate for an 85% detection rate for individual screening tests (data from Wald et al.)[15]
Screening test	False positive rate (%)
First trimester:	
Nuchal translucency	15.0
Combined	4.3
Second trimester:	
Double	13.0
Triple	9.3
Quadruple	6.2
Both trimesters:	
Serum integrated	3.9
Integrated	0.9

Table 1.7 Odds of an affected pregnancy, and procedure-related loss rate of unaffected pregnancies according to type of screening test. (Adapted from Wald et al.)[15]

Screening test	Odds of affected pregnancy for a screen-positive result	Procedure-related unaffected fetal losses/100 000 women screened
First trimester:		
Nuchal translucency	1:94	108
Combined	1:22	35
Second trimester:		
Double	1:68	94
Triple	1:49	67
Quadruple	1:32	45
Both trimesters:		
Serum integrated	1:20	28
Integrated	1:5	6

study in Table 1.6 are given for 11 completed weeks of gestation.

The design of the SURUSS study has made comparison between different first- and second-trimester screening programmes possible.[15] No interventions took place until after collection of the second-trimester samples. Down syndrome pregnancies and pregnancies with abnormal screening markers are at increased risk of spontaneous fetal loss. This means that the screening performance of first-trimester tests in comparison with second-trimester tests tends to be overestimated, since a number of affected pregnancies that would have miscarried spontaneously, and therefore remained unidentified, are detected.

A comparison of the false-positive rates, for a fixed detection rate of 85%, for the different screening options is illustrated in Table 1.6. The integrated test was the most effective screening test, with a false-positive rate of 0.9% for an 85% detection rate. The odds of a screen-positive pregnancy actually being affected by Down syndrome are shown in Table 1.7. This table also presents the figures for unaffected fetal losses resulting from prenatal diagnosis for the different screening regimens.

In the SURUSS study, nuchal translucency measurements were not obtained in 9% of women during a 20-minute examination. The screening performance of nuchal translucency measurements is highest between 10 and 11 weeks of gestation.[16] The performance of serum markers varies with gestation: PAPP-A becomes less discriminatory as gestation advances, whereas free βhCG becomes more discriminatory.

In this analysis, the integrated test was the test of choice. If nuchal translucency measurement is not available, the serum integrated test is the next best option. The quadruple test is the preferred option for women presenting for the first time in the second trimester. For women wishing information before 14 weeks of gestation the combined test is best.

CONTINGENT SCREENING

With contingent screening, all women are offered a combined first-trimester test and, on the basis of the result, are stratified into one of three groups:

- high risk-positive – offered a diagnostic test
- screen negative – no further testing
- intermediate risk-positive – proceed to the integrated test.

The FaSTER trial provides data for contingent screening for Down syndrome.[17] This involved first-trimester nuchal translucency and concurrent maternal serum samples, followed by further serum markers in the second trimester. Women whose fetuses had a septated cystic hygroma on scan were offered immediate prenatal diagnosis. The process was:

1. Nuchal translucency, PAPP-A, free βhCG at 11–13 weeks of gestation.
2. First-trimester risk greater than 1/30 – high risk: prenatal diagnosis offered.
3. First-trimester risk less than 1/1500 – screen negative: no further action.
4. First-trimester risk greater than 1/30–1500 – intermediate risk: proceed to AFP, hCG uE_3 and inhibin at 15–18 weeks.
5. Second-trimester risk greater than 1/270 – offered prenatal diagnosis.

In this study, the detection rate for contingent screening was 91% for a 4.5% false positive rate.

SEQUENTIAL SCREENING

In sequential screening, all women are offered a first-trimester combined test. Those identified as high risk are offered diagnostic testing. All of the remaining women proceed to the integrated test in the second trimester: that is, first-trimester combined markers are integrated with second-trimester serum markers as discussed previously.

COMPARISON OF THE THREE MODELS

With contingent and sequential screening, there is disclosure of an intermediate result. For these two screening programmes to perform effectively, a risk cut-off point of 1/30 or higher is needed to achieve a low enough false-positive rate for the first-trimester step of testing. It has been calculated that, for a detection rate of 90%, the false-positive rate of integrated, sequential and contingent screening is 2.15%, 2.25% and 2.42%, respectively.[18]

Factors to consider when comparing the three models of testing

- Integrated testing achieves the lowest false-positive rate for a given detection rate and is associated with lower procedure-related loss rates of unaffected fetuses.
- Sequential and contingent screening label women as being at high or low risk on the basis of limited information.
- Sequential and contingent screening will identify 66% of affected pregnancies by the end of the first trimester, allowing earlier termination of pregnancy. Some of these first-trimester pregnancies would have miscarried spontaneously, avoiding the distressing decision to opt for pregnancy termination. It has been estimated that approximately 23% of Down syndrome pregnancies miscarry between the time of amniocentesis and term.[19]
- The intermediate positive risk group in the contingent screening programme will receive two different risks. A low risk result from the second-trimester part of the test may not be sufficient to allay the anxiety generated by a higher-risk first-trimester result.
- In contrast to contingent and sequential screening, the integrated screening test treats all women in the same way and a single risk is generated on the basis of all the screening information.

First-trimester versus second-trimester screening

One of the main reasons for developing first-trimester screening options has been the perceived advantage that earlier detection of chromosomal abnormalities and, hence, earlier termination of pregnancy by a surgical method is less emotionally traumatic for the woman. Whether or not this is the case, and obviously individual women will feel differently about this part of their care, certain aspects of first-trimester screening should be considered.

There is a natural attrition rate for aneuploid pregnancies as gestation advances and thus first-trimester screening will identify a proportion of pregnancies that were destined to miscarry spontaneously. This criticism obviously also applies to second-trimester programmes but the rate of fetal lethality is higher between the time of chorionic villus sampling (CVS) and term (43%) compared with the time of amniocentesis and term (23%).[19] There is evidence to indicate that the fetal lethality in cases of trisomy 21 is higher in those fetuses with the biggest nuchal translucency measurements, demonstrating that this ultrasound marker will detect a number of pregnancies that would otherwise miscarry spontaneously. Thus, the potential advantage of earlier termination of pregnancy has to be weighed against the fact that first-trimester screening will 'convert' a proportion of spontaneous miscarriages to pregnancy terminations and the psychological impact of this factor needs to be considered.

CVS is the diagnostic procedure for karyotyping in the first trimester. It is technically more demanding than amniocentesis and, in general, a higher procedure-related loss rate is reported (1–2% compared with 0.5–1.0%). Also, the rate of mosaicism is higher with CVS, necessitating a subsequent amniocentesis in a small proportion of pregnancies.

Women who have had a karyotypically abnormal pregnancy are traditionally offered diagnostic testing in subsequent pregnancies. As discussed above, first-trimester screening will permit the identification of a number of aneuploid pregnancies that were destined to miscarry spontaneously, following which karyotyping would not be a routine issue in future pregnancies. Therefore, first-trimester screening will identify a group of women who will be faced with decisions regarding prenatal diagnostic testing in future pregnancies who would not have been identified by a second-trimester programme.

Other first-trimester ultrasound markers of aneuploidy

NASAL BONE

Absent or hypoplastic nasal bone is a feature of trisomy 21. The fetal nasal bone can be identified on ultrasound from 11 weeks of gestation by obtaining a mid-sagittal image of the fetal profile. Absence of the nasal bone has been reported in 60–73% of cases of trisomy 21 and 0.2–1.0% of normal fetuses.[20–23] In chromosomally normal fetuses, absent nasal bone is related to ethnicity (Afro-Caribbean 9%, white 2.2%, Asian 5%); crown–rump length (the frequency of absence falls with increasing crown–rump length) and nuchal translucency (the frequency of absence is higher with increasing nuchal translucency measurements). Incorporation of absent nasal bone into first-trimester combined screening using nuchal translucency and serum markers could improve trisomy 21 detection rates to 97%, for a 5% false-positive rate. These data are from specialist centres and may not be reproducible in the general population. Large studies are required to determine feasibility. Absent nasal bone is also a feature of other chromosomal abnormalities: trisomy 18, 57.1%; trisomy 13, 31.8%; Turner syndrome, 8.8%.[24]

DUCTUS VENOSUS

There should be forward flow in the ductus venosus throughout the cardiac cycle. Reversed flow during atrial contraction can be associated with cardiac abnormalities and aneuploidy. Abnormal ductus venosus flow velocities have been reported in 59–93% of aneuploid fetuses, in contrast to 3–21% of euploid fetuses.[4,25] As with examination of the nasal bone, ductus venosus assessment requires time and skill and is unlikely to be part of the routine risk assessment for aneuploidy.

SECOND-TRIMESTER ULTRASOUND AND ANEUPLOIDY

The association between structural anomalies and abnormal karyotype is well recognised. Detection of a structural anomaly on scan must prompt a full detailed survey of the fetal anatomy for the presence of additional defects, since the risk of aneuploidy increases in the presence of multiple abnormalities. Structural defects associated with trisomies 21, 18 and 13 are illustrated in Table 1.8.

Congenital heart disease (CHD) is the most common abnormality in trisomy 21 and it is present in 40–45% of cases. Atrioventricular canal defects are most frequent (45%) and ventricular septal defects are the next most common cardiac anomaly (35%). When duodenal atresia is detected on antenatal ultrasound, trisomy 21 is present in approximately 30% of cases. The majority (80–86%) of fetuses with trisomy 18 will have features amenable to ultrasound diagnosis. The most common finding is fetal growth restriction, which is present in 89% of affected fetuses scanned after 24 weeks of gestation. Eighty to ninety percent of trisomy 18 cases will have CHD, ventricular septal defect being most frequent. Prenatal ultrasound diagnosis of trisomy 13 is possible in 90–100% of cases. Eighty to ninety percent of cases have CHD, with ventricular septal

Table 1.8   Structural anomalies associated with trisomies 21, 18 and 13

Trisomy 21	Trisomy 18	Trisomy 13
Congenital heart disease (AV canal defect)	Fetal growth restriction	Congenital heart disease (VSD)
Duodenal atresia	Congenital heart disease (VSD)	Holoprosencephaly
Exomphalos	Exomphalos	Midline facial defects
Tracheo-oesophageal fistula	Congenital diaphragmatic hernia	Renal anomalies
Cystic hygroma	Rockerbottom feet	Exomphalos
Hydrothorax	Clenched fists with overlapping index finger	Neural tube defects
Ventriculomegaly		Polydactyly
		Fetal growth restriction

VSD = ventricular septal defect

defect again being most common. Central nervous system abnormalities are more frequent in trisomy 13. Holoprosencephaly is reported in 30–40% of cases. Renal anomalies are present in one-third and include multicystic kidney disease and ureteric obstruction. Fetal growth restriction will be seen in 50% of fetuses with trisomy 13.[26,27]

Not all fetuses with aneuploidy will have major structural anomalies and, hence, are not amenable to detection by second-trimester ultrasound. This is particularly true for trisomy 21, in which only 30–50% of affected fetuses in the general obstetric population are detected by ultrasound features. As a result, exploration of the role of soft markers as a means of improving detection has been the subject of much discussion in the literature. Soft markers are discussed in Chapter 3. There are a number of important points to consider regarding soft markers:

- they are ultrasound features that are variants of normal and in themselves may not be pathological
- they are present in up to 15% of otherwise normal mid-trimester pregnancies
- the original data presented regarding their significance was obtained in high-risk populations and cannot be routinely applied to the general population
- the majority of women described in the original data discussing soft markers had not had any form of screening and certainly not first-trimester screening
- with the advent of first-trimester screening, up to 90% of cases of trisomy 21 will be identified before the second-trimester scan. As a result, the fetuses found to have soft markers in the second trimester are more likely to be karyotypically normal than those identified in the pre-screening era.

Screening in multiple pregnancy

Multiple pregnancy is associated with a higher risk of chromosomal abnormality than singleton pregnancy. The risk is largely determined by the zygosity of the pregnancy. Monozygotic twins that follow splitting of a single fertilised ovum are almost always genetically identical. Very rarely, monozygotic twins will have discordant genetic material, hence both sacs should be sampled for genetic diagnosis. Dizygotic twins result from fertilisation of separate ova, resulting in genetically distinct individuals, and chromosomal abnormalities in dizygotic twins are generally discordant.

First-trimester chorionicity is the most accurate method for establishing zygosity in multiple pregnancies (Chapter 9). In general, monochorionic twins are monozygotic. There are reports of dizygotic twins with monochorionic placentation following assisted conception but this situation is very rare. Dichorionic twins can be dizygotic or monozygotic, depending on when the fertilised ovum splits. Given that there are twice as many dizygous as monozygous twin pregnancies, the majority of dichorionic twin pregnancies (90%), but not all, will be dizygous.

In monozygotic twin pregnancies, the maternal age-related risk of chromosomal abnormality for each fetus is the same as for a singleton pregnancy. In a dizygotic twin pregnancy, each twin has an independent maternal age-related risk for aneuploidy and so the chance of at least one fetus being affected is approximately twice as high as an equivalent singleton pregnancy.

CONSIDERATIONS

Chromosomal anomalies in non-identical (dizygous) twin pregnancies are likely to be discordant. Prenatal diagnosis and selective termination of an affected fetus poses risk to the unaffected fetus. As a result, decision making regarding prenatal screening is complex in the setting of multiple pregnancy.

Any form of screening that includes maternal serum markers can only give a pregnancy-specific risk, not a fetus-specific risk. Thus, for dizygotic twins, biochemical screening will not differentiate the risk for each individual fetus. Experience with maternal serum screening in twin pregnancies is limited. On average, the serum markers are twice as high as for singletons of equivalent gestational age. However, there is the risk that where discordant anomaly exists, levels from the affected fetus will be brought closer to the mean by the levels of the unaffected twin.

Mathematical models have been constructed to predict risk on the basis of biochemical screening in twin pregnancies. A detection rate of 51% (for a false-positive rate of 5%) using second-trimester βhCG and AFP has been quoted.[28] However, mathematical modelling may be an oversimplification. It is also recognised that assisted conception, likely to be responsible for a number of multiple pregnancies, may affect analyte levels. Owing to the paucity of data, biochemical screening is not routinely offered in the majority of centres.

Nuchal translucency is an anatomical measurement that can obtained for each fetus and therefore used to assign a fetus-specific risk of aneuploidy. Nuchal translucency distribution in twin pregnancies is not significantly different from that of singletons. Detection rates of 88% (for a false-positive rate of 7.3%) are possible.[29] The prevalence of increased nuchal translucency is higher in monochorionic twins and may be an early indicator of twin–twin transfusion syndrome.

As discussed before, combined first-trimester screening, because it includes biochemistry, will only generate a pregnancy-specific risk in the case of dizygotic twins. A detection rate of 75% for a false-positive rate of 9% has been achieved.[30] However, this requires further prospective study before it is applied routinely to the general population.

Parents must be very clear about what they are embarking upon when pursuing screening in a multiple pregnancy. An anatomical marker (nuchal translucency) has the advantage that it will generate a fetus-specific risk, which is not possible when biochemistry is included. Diagnostic testing requires that both fetuses are sampled, either by CVS or amniocentesis (occasionally monozygotic twins have a different genetic makeup). Options for prenatal diagnosis may be limited to amniocentesis if there is no certainty that each placenta can be sampled separately. Procedure-related loss risks are higher with multiple sampling and then there are the risks associated with selective reduction, including the psychological sequelae of loss of the entire pregnancy, which is a potential complication.

Summary

There have been major advances in screening programmes for trisomy 21 in recent years. The various options have their advantages and disadvantages. Women will differ in their priorities around prenatal screening. Some will wish information at the earliest opportunity, whereas as others will want the test that has the lowest false-positive rate and, hence, the lowest risk of procedure-related loss of an unaffected pregnancy with subsequent diagnostic testing. Irrespective of the method of screening, it is vital that women receive the correct information so that they can decide whether or not prenatal screening is something they wish to take up and that, should they do so, they are fully aware of its implications.

References

1. Wald NJ, Kennard A, Hackshaw A, McGuire A. Antenatal screening for Down's syndrome. *J Med Screen* 1997;4:181–246.

2. Wald NJ, Rodeck C, Hackshaw AJ, Walters J, Chitty L, Mackinson AM. First and second trimester antenatal screening for Down's syndrome: the results of the Serum, Urine and Ultrasound Screening Study (SURUSS). *J Med Screen* 2003;10:56–104.

3. Crossley JA, Aitken DA, Connor JM. Second trimester unconjugated oestriol levels in maternal serum from chromosomally abnormal pregnancies using an optimized assay. *Prenat Diagn* 1993;13:271–80.

4. Malone FD, Canick JA, Ball RH, Nyberg DA, Comstock CH, Bukowski R, *et al.* First-trimester or second-trimester screening, or both, for Down's syndrome. *N Engl J Med* 2005;353:2001–11.

5. Wald NJ, Huttly WJ. Rudnicka AR. Prenatal screening for Down syndrome: the problem of recurrent false-positives. *Prenat Diagn* 2004;24:389-92.

6. Wald NJ, Barnes IM, Birger R, Huttly W. Effect on Down syndrome screening performance of adjusting for marker levels in a previous pregnancy. *Prenat Diagn* 2006;26:539–44.

7. Krantz DA, Larsen JW, Buchanan PD, Macri JN. First-trimester Down syndrome screening: Free β-human chorionic gonadotrophin and pregnancy-associated plasma protein A. *Am J Obstet Gynecol* 1996;174:612–16.

8. Wald NJ, George L, Smith D, Densem JW, Petterson K. Serum screening for Down's syndrome between 8 and 14 weeks of pregnancy. *Br J Obstet Gynaecol* 1996;103:407–12.

9. Snijders RJM, Noble P, Sebire N, Souka A, Nicolaides KH. UK multicentre project on assessment of risk of trisomy 21 by maternal age and fetal nuchal translucency thickness at 10-14 weeks gestation. *Lancet* 1998;351:343–6.

10. Atzei A, Gajewska K, Huggon IC, Allan L, Nicolaides KH. Relationship between nuchal translucency thickness and prevalence of major cardiac defects in fetuses with normal karyotype. *Ultrasound Obstet Gynecol* 2005;26:154–7.

11. Souka AP, Von Kaisenberg CS, Hyett JA, Sonek JD, Nicolaides KH. Increased nuchal translucency with normal karyotype. *Am J Obstet Gynecol* 1999;192:1005–21.

12. Wald NJ, Hackshaw AK. Combining ultrasound and biochemistry in first-trimester screening for Down's syndrome. *Prenat Diagn* 1997;17:821–9.

13. Spencer K, Souter V, Tul N, Snijders R, Nicolaides KH. A screening programme for trisomy 21 at 10-14 weeks using fetal nuchal translucency, maternal serum free β-human chorionic gonadotrophin and pregnancy associated plasma protein-A. *Ultrasound Obstet Gynecol* 1999;13:231–7.

14. Dunstan FDJ, Nix ABJ. Screening for Down's syndrome: the effect of test date on the detection rate. *Ann Clin Biochem* 1998;35:57–61.

15. Wald NJ, Rodeck C, Hackshaw AK, Rudnicka A. SURUSS in perspective. *BJOG* 2004;111:521–31.

16. Wald N, Rodeck C, Rudnicka A, Hackshaw A. Nuchal translucency and gestational age. *Prenat Diagn* 2004;24:150–3.

17. Cuckle HS, Malone FD, Wright D, Porter TF, Nyberg DA, Comstock CH, *et al.* Contingent screening for Down syndrome: results from the FaSTER trial. *Prenat Diagn* 2008;8:89–94.

18. Wald NJ, Rudnicka AR, Bestwick JP. Sequential and contingent prenatal screening for Down syndrome. *Prenat Diagn* 2006;26:769–77.

19. Morris JK, Wald NJ, Watt HC. Fetal loss in Down syndrome pregnancies. *Prenat Diagn* 1999;19:142–5.

20. Cicero S, Curcio P, Papageorghiu A, Sonek J, Nicolaides K. Absence of nasal bone in fetuses with trisomy 21 at 11–14 weeks' gestation: an observational study. *Lancet* 2001;358:1665–7.

21. Otano L, Aiello H, Igarzabal L, Matayoshi T, Gadow EC. Association between first trimester absence of fetal nasal bone on ultrasound and Down's syndrome. *Prenat Diagn* 2002;22:930–2.

22. Orlandi F, Bilardo CM, Campogrande M, Krantz D, Hallahan T, Rossi C, *et al.* Measurement of nasal bone length at 11–14 weeks of pregnancy and its potential role in Down syndrome risk assessment. *Ultrasound Obstet Gynecol* 2003;22:36–9.

23. Cicero S, Rembouskos G, Vandecruys H, Hogg M, Nicolaides KH. Likelihood ratio for trisomy 21 in fetuses with absent nasal bone at the 11–14 week scan. *Ultrasound Obstet Gynecol* 2004;23:218–23.

24. Cicero S, Longo D, Rembouskos G, Sacchini C, Nicolaides KH. Absent nasal bone at 11–14 weeks gestation and chromosomal defects. *Ultrasound Obstet Gynecol* 2003;22:31–5.

25. Brigatti KW, Malone FD. First-trimester screening for aneuploidy. *Obstet Gynecol Clin N Am* 2004;31:1–20.

26. Stewart TL. Screening for aneuploidy: the genetic sonogram. *Obstet Gynecol Clin N Am* 2004;31:21–33.

27. Shipp TD, Benacerraf BR. Second trimester ultrasound screening for chromosomal abnormalities. *Prenat Diagn* 2002;22:296–307.

28. Spencer K, Salonen R, Muller F. Down's syndrome screening in multiple pregnancies using alpha-fetoprotein and free beta hCG. *Prenat Diagn* 1994;14:537–42.

29. Sebire NJ, Snijders RJM, Hughes K, Sepulveda W, Nicolaides KH. Screening for trisomy 21 in twin pregnancies by maternal age and fetal nuchal translucency thickness at 10-14 weeks gestation. *Br J Obstet Gynaecol* 1996;103:999–1003.

30. Spencer K, Nicolaides KH. Screening for trisomy 21 in twins using first trimester ultrasound and maternal serum biochemistry in a one-stop clinic: a review of three years experience. *BJOG* 2003;110:276–80.

31. Connor M, Ferguson-Smith M, editors. *Essential Medical Genetics.* 5th ed. Oxford: Blackwell Science; 1997.

2 Prenatal diagnostic techniques

Introduction

Antenatal screening identifies those pregnancies at 'high risk' of fetal complications, such as aneuploidy, intrauterine infection and fetal anaemia, but the diagnosis can only be confirmed or refuted by direct examination of fetal tissue or blood. Until recently, fetal cells could only be obtained by an invasive procedure: amniocentesis, chorionic villus sampling (CVS) or cordocentesis. While fetal cells can now be extracted from the maternal circulation and analysed for specific indications, this technique is not widely available and it clinical use remains limited. Invasive testing therefore remains the cornerstone of prenatal diagnosis.

This chapter will focus on the prenatal diagnostic techniques used to determine fetal karyotype. Readers are referred to Chapters 5 and 10 for information on the role of prenatal diagnostic tests in the management of fetal anaemia and intrauterine infection.

Who should be offered invasive prenatal testing?

All pregnant women should be made aware that both diagnostic and screening tests for aneuploidy are available in pregnancy. The majority of women will choose to have a screening test, as this carries no innate risk to the pregnancy, and will not wish to discuss diagnostic testing in any form. For others, the consequences of having a child affected by aneuploidy are of such enormity that no screening test will give sufficient reassurance. If such concerns are expressed, the mother must have ample opportunity to discuss the full range of diagnostic tests that are available. It is for the woman to decide which risk is most acceptable.

There are several groups of women at increased risk of aneuploidy in pregnancy who must be made aware of the risks they carry. With this information, they can balance the risk of a problem in the fetus against the risk of a procedure and make an informed decision on whether to proceed with testing or not:

- women who are screen positive
- families with specific chromosome markers
- ultrasound abnormalities identified during pregnancy.

WOMEN WHO ARE SCREEN-POSITIVE

As outlined in Chapter 1, a proportion of pregnancies screened for aneuploidy will be classed as 'high risk'. Those classed as high risk need ample opportunity to discuss their individual risk calculation and the diagnostic tests appropriate for their gestational age.

FAMILIES WITH SPECIFIC CHROMOSOME MARKERS

Women or their partners who carry a balanced chromosome inversion or translocation and are themselves unaffected are at increased risk of chromosome abnormalities in pregnancy. The genetics team should assess these couples to ensure that the correct risk is calculated, the possible outcomes are understood and the correct diagnostic test is offered.

ULTRASOUND ABNORMALITIES IDENTIFIED DURING PREGNANCY

Structural abnormalities in a fetus, such as duodenal atresia, congenital diaphragmatic hernia, cardiac abnormalities, cystic hygroma or holoprosencephaly, are strongly associated with specific chromosome abnormalities. The risks of aneuploidy will vary, depending on the abnormality identified.

Diagnostic tests available in pregnancy

To make an informed decision about prenatal invasive testing, women should be given an outline of all the procedures available, the timing of each test and the pregnancy risks associated with each technique, as outlined in the remainder of this chapter. Ideally, these discussions should be supplemented with explanatory booklets that outline the pertinent points and salient statistics. Informed, written consent should be obtained before any testing is performed.

AMNIOCENTESIS

Technique

Amniocentesis is an ultrasound-guided procedure. Having confirmed fetal viability, an accessible pool of amniotic fluid should be identified. Ideally, passage through the placenta should be avoided but, if this is not achievable, a transplacental approach may be employed. If a transplacental tap is necessary, the thinnest portion of placenta, avoiding the cord insertion point, should be selected.[1]

Using an aseptic technique, a 20- or 22-gauge needle is inserted into the amniotic fluid under continuous ultrasound guidance. The tip of the operator's needle should be visible throughout the procedure (Figure

2.1a,b).[1] This reduces the incidence of bloodstained samples and should prevent damage to the fetus or the umbilical cord. Following removal of the inner stilette, 15–17 ml of amniotic fluid is aspirated before the needle is removed from the uterus.

All women should have their blood group checked either before or at the time of amniocentesis. Those who are rhesus D-negative require 250 iu of anti-D immunoglobulin to prevent rhesus isoimmunisation.[2]

Complications

The major hazard of amniocentesis is pregnancy loss. The loss rate was previously derived from a single-centre, randomised study of amniocentesis that was published in 1986.[3] To date, this is the only truly randomised study that evaluates a prenatal diagnostic technique. The study involved over 4600 women, regarded as at low risk, who were randomised into a 'no amniocentesis' and an 'amniocentesis' group. Amniocentesis was performed using a standard 20-gauge needle technique. The procedure-related fetal loss rate in this group was approximately 1% higher than the loss rate in the 'no-amniocentesis' group. This figure of 1% fetal loss is still widely used when counselling women for amniocentesis.

More recently, several large studies have suggested that the loss rate for mid-trimester amniocentesis is significantly less than 1%. The FaSTER (First- and Second-Trimester Evaluation of Risk for aneuploidy) group reported fetal loss rates following amniocentesis of 1:1600.[4] While the methodology of this report was heavily criticised and the published results therefore questioned, a subsequent meta-analysis[5] and a large single centre review[6] have also reported procedure-related loss rates of less than 1% (0.6–0.14%; 1/300–1/700). As a result of this increasing body of evidence, it is now generally accepted that in centres with appropriately trained staff, performing a large number of procedures, the loss rate following amniocentesis is around 1/200–1/300 and may be lower.

Other, less common, complications that may occur following amniocentesis include vaginal spotting or loss of amniotic fluid. These occur in 1–2% of cases. Spontaneous loss of amniotic fluid following amniocentesis was assumed to result in either miscarriage or a poor fetal outcome but, in most cases, the fluid loss ceases spontaneously, amniotic fluid reaccumulates and a good pregnancy outcome ensues. Very rarely, intrauterine infection will develop, with the rapid onset of generalised sepsis. This necessitates urgent delivery of the pregnancy, irrespective of the gestational age. In routine mid-trimester amniocentesis without spontaneous loss of liquor, the risk of chorioamnionitis is extremely small (1/1000). Prophylactic antibiotics are not indicated and the woman is simply advised to report any unexplained fever or significant pain.

There is no evidence that mid-trimester amniocentesis carried out

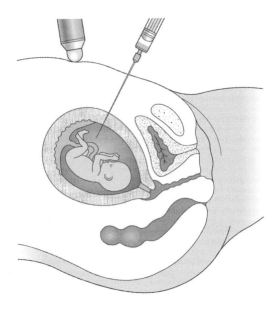

(a)

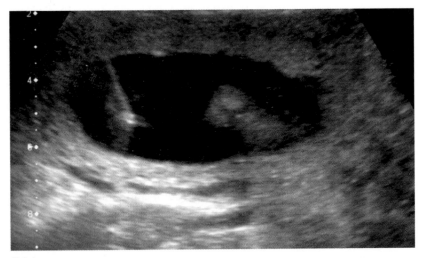

(b)

Figure 2.1 Amniocentesis: (a) diagrammatic view; (b) Transabdominal ultrasound image of the needle-tip visible within a good pocket of amniotic fluid

between 15 and 21 weeks of gestation is associated with risks of fetal abnormality. In particular, there is no significant risk of orthopaedic problems such as talipes.

Timing

Genetic amniocentesis is traditionally offered between 15–20 weeks of gestation. This allows time for the fetal cells to be analysed and, in the event of an abnormal result, time for the couple to proceed with termination of pregnancy, avoiding the need for feticide.

In an attempt to offer the option of earlier testing, amniocentesis between 11 and 14 weeks of gestation has also been evaluated. The Canadian Early and Mid-trimester Amniocentesis Trial (CEMAT) randomly allocated women to early (11–12 weeks plus 6 days) or mid-trimester (15–16 weeks plus 6 days) amniocentesis.[7] This large study highlighted an increased fetal loss rate for early as opposed to mid-trimester amniocentesis (7.6% compared with 5.9% total fetal loss rates), an increase in talipes in the early amniocentesis group (1.3% compared with 0.1%) and an increased incidence of amniotic fluid leakage (3.5% compared with 1.7%). There was also a greater number of culture failures in the early amniocentesis group. For these reasons, the most recent systematic review has concluded that early amniocentesis is not a safe alternative; genetic amniocentesis should only be performed after 14 completed weeks of gestation.[8]

Cytogenetic analysis

Amniocyte culture remains the gold standard for karyotype analysis. Amniotic fluid samples are cultured over a period of 10–14 days. At this point, the amniocytes are arrested during the metaphase stage of cell division, harvested, fixed on a slide and stained with dye. The visible chromosomes are then examined under the microscope. It may take up to 21 days to obtain a final report on the chromosome complement. In addition to aneuploidy, examination of cultured amniocytes should also identify chromosome inversions, deletions and rearrangements.

Occasionally during amniocyte culture, two or more cell lines, each with a different karyotype, may be seen to arise from the same pregnancy fluid. This is known as a mosaic result. When this is found in only one colony of cultured cells, it is usually an *in vitro* error. Where different cell lines are found in multiple colonies, there is the risk of true fetal mosaicism and additional tests are required.

To reduce the time delay in obtaining results for already anxious parents, newer techniques have been introduced (Box 2.1). Fluorescence *in situ* hybridisation (FISH) and quantitative fluorescence polymerase chain reaction (QFPCR) allow rapid evaluation of a small, selected

BOX 2.1   RAPID TESTS FOR KARYOTYPE ANALYSIS

FISH

- Following amniocentesis, fluorescence-labelled DNA probes for areas on chromosome 21, 13 and 18 (± sex chromosomes) are mixed with the uncultured amniocytes.
- When the nuclei are then examined using a fluorescence microscope, normal cells will have two fluorescent spots while, in trisomic cells, three fluorescent spots will be identified.
- Although a result can be obtained within 24–72 hours, the process is very expensive and labour intensive.

QFPCR

- Uncultured amniocytes from 1–2ml of amniotic fluid are collected and the DNA extracted.
- Chromosome-specific, short tandem repeats of DNA from selected chromosomes are then amplified using fluorescence markers.
- Using an automated scanner, the intensity of fluorescence present for each short tandem repeat is quantified and the number of chromosome alleles derived.
- As the technique is automated, a large number of samples can be processed efficiently and the result reported with 48 hours.

number of chromosomes or chromosome markers but these techniques do not routinely identify more complex anomalies in the chromosome complement.

While FISH and QFPCR offer a rapid diagnosis of trisomy or sex-chromosome abnormalities, other chromosome problems, such as rearrangements or deletions, will not be detected unless additional probes are specifically requested. For this reason, many laboratories still offer a full amniocyte culture report in addition to any rapid tests provided.

CHORIONIC VILLUS SAMPLING

The technique of CVS was first described as a means of first-trimester sex-chromosome determination in China.[9] It was introduced into the West by a team at St Mary's Hospital in London and was subsequently developed during the late 1980s in Europe and America.

Technique

Most of the early trials of CVS relied on transcervical sampling but the transabdominal route has now become the technique of choice. This route is preferred by women, has a lower rate of immediate complications, a lower risk of intrauterine infection and a shorter learning curve. The transcervical route may still be used when there is a low-lying posterior

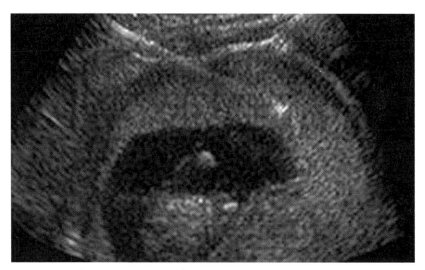

Figure 2.2 Ultrasound image of the needle inserted into the placenta during chorionic villus sampling

placenta. The remainder of this section will focus on transabdominal CVS.

Several modifications have been described for transabdominal CVS. These all perform equally well in experienced hands and the selection of technique used is therefore determined primarily by operator experience.

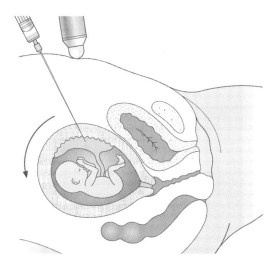

Figure 2.3 Chorionic villus biopsy of an anterior placenta, in which needle is intentionally inserted into placenta

The placental position should be localised and seen to be accessible without entry into the gestation sac. A full bladder, which will usually push the uterus into an axial or slightly retroverted position, may facilitate access to an anterior placenta (Figure 2.2). Sampling a posterior placenta will generally be helped by asking the patient to empty her bladder, as the uterus adopts a more anteverted position (Figure 2.3).

If local anaesthesia is used, this should be inserted under ultrasound guidance, through the abdominal wall to the level of the myometrium. Thereafter, an 18-gauge needle is progressively inserted through the layers of the abdominal wall and the myometrium until the placenta is entered (Figure 2.4). Suction is applied via the aspirating syringe and the needle and attached syringe moved five to ten times within the placental tissue. Following aspiration, the needle and attached syringe are removed and the sample injected directly into culture medium. The sample must be examined to ensure that a sufficient number of chorionic villi are present. If the sample is inadequate, the whole procedure must be repeated with reinsertion of the 18-gauge needle.

An alternative approach is to use a 'double-needle' technique. The 18-gauge needle, once in the myometrium, is used as a 'guide' needle and a smaller 20- or 21-gauge needle inserted through the shaft. Thereafter, suction is applied via the aspirating syringe and the inner needle and syringe are moved in the placental tissue five to ten times. The 20-gauge needle and attached syringe alone are removed and the sample is injected into culture medium. If the sample is inadequate, the 20-gauge needle may be reinserted several times, through the guide needle, until sufficient villi are identified, thus avoiding the need to reinsert a large-gauge needle.

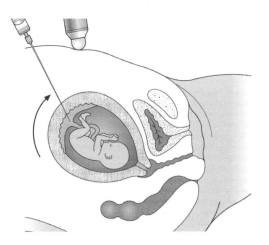

Figure 2.4 Chorionic villus biopsy of a posterior placenta

In some centres, the aspirating syringe and needle are partially filled with sterile saline to aid aspiration of villus material.

Irrespective of the technique used, it is suggested that, in experienced hands, an adequate sample should be obtained with one 18-gauge needle insertion in 95% of cases.

All women who are RhD-negative who have not been immunised must have anti-D immunoglobulin 250 iu administered intramuscularly following the procedure.[2]

Complications

As with amniocentesis, the greatest risk of CVS is pregnancy loss. The initial experience of CVS suggested the pregnancy loss rate to be at least 1% and up to 4%, greater than the loss rate associated with amniocentesis. As a result, there was little demand for the procedure. Recent experience of CVS is more favourable. A systematic review of studies found the loss rate following transabdominal CVS to be almost identical to the loss rate following mid-trimester amniocentesis (0.7%).[5] As with all invasive techniques, it is likely that the loss rate is much higher in less experienced hands.

In addition to fetal loss, several centres reported in the early 1990s an association with limb reduction defects. This was presumed to be due to placental microembolisation occurring at the time of the procedure. A World Health Organization statement, following an analysis of 80 000 cases of CVS performed from 8 completed weeks onwards, failed to confirm these earlier findings but, in light of these risks, genetic CVS is now usually performed beyond 10 weeks of gestation.

Contraindications

Transabdominal CVS may be impossible to carry out if there are obstacles to the safe passage of the sampling needle, such as bowel attached to the abdominal wall or multiple fibroids. Transcervical CVS should not be carried out in the presence of vaginal or cervical infection. With either route, it is wise to postpone the investigation if there is active bleeding suggestive of a possible threatened miscarriage.

Timing

The accepted gestational age for genetic CVS is between 10 and 12 weeks of gestation. The placenta at this stage of pregnancy is easy to identify and of such thickness that safe sampling is usually possible. Although CVS can be carried out at later stages of pregnancy, second-trimester amniocentesis is generally preferred, because the technique is technically more straightforward, is deemed less uncomfortable for the woman and has a lower rate of mosaic results.

Cytogenetic analysis

The CVS sample is manually prepared, leaving clean chorionic villi for analysis. The sample is then either reported directly (a rapid result) or cultured before analysis.

A rapid result is obtained by examining cytotrophoblastic cells arrested in metaphase and a result usually available within 24–48 hours. A standard culture normally takes 10–15 days, after which time the mesenchymal cells are harvested and standard chromosome preparations obtained. Direct reports are associated with a small false-negative and false-positive risk and most laboratories therefore proceed with a full long-term culture to validate any preliminary or rapid reports.

CVS diagnosis is only possible on the assumption that the chromosome complement of the fetus and chorionic tissue are identical. This is true for the vast majority of pregnancies but, occasionally, different cell lines are found in the fetus and placenta, a condition known as confined placental mosaicism. This condition occurs in 1–2% of all CVS samples and necessitates further testing in the pregnancy. True mosaicism, the presence of two or more cell lines within one fetus is extremely rare.

As with amniocentesis, QFPCR and FISH (Box 2.1) are now used to speed up the diagnosis of aneuploidy in CVS specimens. Chorionic villi are also suitable for investigations other than cytogenetic analyses: the tissue is metabolically active and can thus be used in the diagnosis of many inherited metabolic diseases. The amount of DNA obtained from a conventional sample allows for many analyses using recombinant DNA technology. Such analyses are not usually possible with amniotic fluid cells.

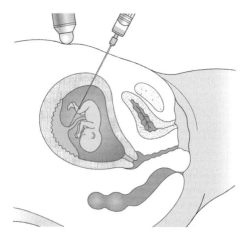

Figure 2.5 Cordocentesis, in which the needle is inserted into the umbilical vein where the umbilical cord joins the placenta

CORDOCENTESIS

Cordocentesis as a method of fetal blood sampling was first carried out in the 1960s under fetoscopic guidance and carried a procedure-related fetal loss rate of over 5%. The first percutaneous umbilical cord sampling under ultrasound control was reported by Daffos *et al.* in 1983.[10] This development revolutionised the technique, allowing access to the fetal vascular compartment for both diagnostic and therapeutic means, with a procedure-related fetal loss rate of less than 2%. Owing to the introduction of FISH and QFPCR, fetal blood sampling is rarely used to test for aneuploidy in current practice but it may be required to evaluate a fetal karyotype if a mosaic result is obtained at the time of CVS or amniocentesis.

Cord blood sampling still has a place in the investigation of fetal infection and the anaemia that can follow infections such as parvovirus, congenital toxoplasmosis and rhesus isoimmunisation.

Technique

The umbilical vein is identified ultrasonically and, using either a biopsy guide or a freehand technique, a 20-gauge spinal needle is inserted under direct ultrasound control (Figure 2.5). The procedure is technically more difficult and the loss rate higher if the procedure is carried out before 20 weeks of gestation. The site of cord insertion at the placenta, where the cord is relatively fixed, is the most favoured target for cordocentesis. Local anaesthesia is not generally used.

Complications

The major complications of cordocentesis are fetal bradycardia, bleeding at the puncture site or occasionally asystole. The world experience of cordocentesis is much smaller than for other invasive techniques such as CVS or amniocentesis but there are some large studies.[11] With modern equipment, the umbilical vein should be successfully punctured in more than 90% of cases. The loss rate in both singleton and multiple pregnancies is around 1.4%.

WHICH PROCEDURE AT WHICH GESTATION?

Transabdominal CVS is the diagnostic technique of choice in pregnancies of less than 15 weeks of gestation. In experienced hands, there is minimal risk of pregnancy loss and failed or mosaic cultures are rare. It remains a technically demanding procedure requiring extensive operator experience to achieve competency. In pregnancies of greater than 15 weeks of gestation, mid-trimester amniocentesis is the preferred procedure. It is technically less complex, has a very low risk of pregnancy loss in experienced hands and has very few additional risks. Owing to the technical limitations and improvements in the speed of cytogenetic analysis, cordo-centesis is now reserved for specific or difficult diagnostic dilemmas.

Diagnostic testing in multiple pregnancy

Diagnostic testing in women with a multiple pregnancy is a complex clinical scenario that raises major ethical dilemmas for parents; in particular, the options for pregnancy management in the event that only one fetus is found to be affected.

AMNIOCENTESIS

The relative location of each gestation sac and placenta must be carefully documented. Although sampling both gestation sacs using a single-needle insertion has been described, there are theoretical concerns about sample mixing, failure to adequately puncture the inter-twin membrane and therefore failure to truly sample both sacs and potential damage to the inter-twin membrane. Many clinicians therefore use a double-needle insertion using the technique previously described for CVS or sample each gestation sac using a separate needle insertion point for each sac. It is critical that the samples obtained are precisely labelled, to ensure that the results can be accurately linked to the correct gestation sac, thus avoiding a fatal error if selective termination is indicated.

There is wide variation in the reported post-procedure loss rate in multiple pregnancies, ranging from 0% to 3% greater than the background rate.

CHORIONIC VILLUS SAMPLING

CVS in a multiple pregnancy is a technically demanding procedure. In a monochorionic twin pregnancy, some parents will request that only one sample is obtained but they must be aware that ultrasound-determined chorionicity may not be 100% accurate. For all other multiple pregnancies, the placental positions must be clearly mapped and documented, to ensure that each placental mass is sampled. In addition, the operator should note whether the bladder is full or empty, as this can significantly alter how each gestation sac and placenta appear to be positioned. Separate needles should be used to prevent cross contamination of the samples. The samples must be labelled in such a way that each result can be matched to the appropriate fetus.

As for amniocentesis, there are limited data available on the loss rate following CVS in multiple pregnancies but it would appear to be no different to the background loss rates for twin pregnancies. There is an increased risk of sampling error and placental mosaicism during CVS in multiple pregnancies. With experienced operators, the risk of sample error is greatly reduced.

Diagnostic testing in women with chronic infection

Women infected with HIV, hepatitis B virus or hepatitis C virus should only proceed with diagnostic testing after a full evaluation of the risks of mother-to-child transmission.[12]

HIV

Before the introduction of antiretroviral therapy, several groups reported mother-to-child transmission rates of up to 30% in women who were HIV-positive undergoing amniocentesis. The majority of these procedures were performed in the third trimester, a period now associated with the highest risk of vertical transmission. As a result, few pregnant women who were HIV-positive were even offered invasive testing. The introduction of antiretroviral therapy during pregnancy has changed the risks of mother-to-child transmission dramatically. Recent reports would suggest that in selected mothers who are HIV infected who are treated with effective antiretroviral therapy, mother-to-child transmission rates are not increased following amniocentesis. Women who are HIV-positive with high HIV viral counts, coexisting hepatitis C infection and/or immunosuppression are at increased risk of mother-to-child transmission and should be discouraged from any invasive testing.

HEPATITIS B

The risk of fetal infection following amniocentesis in women with hepatitis B is low, provided that appropriate immunoprophylaxis is commenced in the newborn period. Those with hepatitis B e antigen have an increased infectivity risk and should be counselled that the risk of mother-to-child transmission is uncertain.

HEPATITIS C

Although there are limited data available, in the absence of comorbidities, hepatitis C does not appear to increase the risk of mother-to-child transmission.

Audit of invasive prenatal diagnostic procedures

It is absolutely vital that units undertaking prenatal diagnostic procedures accurately record the number and type of procedures performed by each operator, any and all procedure-related complications and the outcomes of all pregnancies. Such audits are essential if accurate evaluation of the service is to be provided.

For the future: non-invasive prenatal diagnosis

To be able to offer prenatal diagnostic tests that have no risk to the pregnancy, investigators have tried to isolate fetal cells from the maternal serum. Although this is now technically possible, the small number of cells actually present within maternal serum has prevented this technique from being developed to a clinically useful level.

In 1997, Lo *et al.*[13] identified that portions of fetal DNA, released from the placental syncytiotrophoblast, were present in reasonable quantities within the maternal serum. These cell-free fetal DNA segments are substantially smaller in size than maternal DNA and are therefore distinguishable. They are present in all pregnant women from early in the first trimester and they are cleared from maternal serum within a week of delivery. Their presence in maternal serum opened a new door of opportunity for clinically effective non-invasive prenatal diagnosis.

Owing to the relatively small quantities of fetal DNA in the maternal circulation (approximately 5% of total DNA), it has proved difficult to isolate pure extracts of fetal DNA. Instead, prenatal diagnosis has focused on identifying paternally inherited genes within the DNA pool that will not be present in maternal DNA, such as DNA from the Y chromosome or DNA from the *RHD* gene in a mother who is rhesus negative. As such, non-invasive prenatal diagnosis is frequently one of exclusion (the absence of Y chromosome material implies that the fetus is female) and can therefore only be used confidently in well-defined areas; namely, sex-determination, RhD and other blood group genotyping and specific single-gene disorders, such as β-thalassaemia.

POTENTIAL PROBLEMS

While these developments have proved very promising, there are a few cautionary points to note. Even within the parameters mentioned, no large studies have demonstrated 100% sensitivity and specificity. Parents need to be fully counselled and made aware of the potential pitfalls of a false-negative result. The studies themselves have looked at largely 'at risk' populations and need to be replicated within the general population. In addition, there are ethical dilemmas that need to be addressed: sex determination with a view to sex-selection may be requested for non-medical indications and, with huge commercial input to these developments, there may well be economic pressure from companies to make these tests readily available to the consumer. Currently, there is no formal legislation that covers non-invasive prenatal diagnosis.

FINALLY

The major challenge for those pioneering non-invasive prenatal diagnosis is the detection of fetal aneuploidy. If this proved possible, the majority of invasive prenatal diagnostic tests could be avoided.

To detect aneuploidy, a technique to identify trisomic fetal material needs to be identified. Previous techniques that identify paternally inherited genetic material cannot be used in this situation, so a novel approach is required. The recent discovery of fetal mRNA in maternal serum may prove to be a critical element in this process. If mRNA that is unique to fetal tissue, such as the placenta, can be isolated and the origins of the DNA can be localised to a specific gene (for example, on chromosome 21 or 18 or 13), there is the possibility of determining gene dosage in the fetus and establishing or excluding aneuploidy.

The most promising placental candidate that has been isolated to date is PLAC4 (placenta specific 4) which is located on chromosome 21. While PLAC4 is specific to the fetus and its locus is well-defined, there are still technical difficulties in accurately determining the chromosome dosage represented. However, given the huge commercial backing to this technology, it is likely that a solution will be found in the near future.

Conclusion

Given the rapidly changing face of prenatal diagnosis, it is important that those involved in antenatal care are conversant with the full spectrum of prenatal testing available to ensure that parents are reliably informed of the most appropriate options available to them, including the risks and limitations of each technique. Any invasive procedures performed should be executed with technical competence and minimal risk to the pregnancy. We await the results of continuing research in non-invasive prenatal diagnosis techniques to further refine the shape of prenatal testing offered on a population-wide basis in the next decade.

References

1. Royal College of Obstetricians and Gynaecologists. *Amniocentesis*. Green-top Guideline No. 8. London: RCOG; 2005 [www.rcog.org.uk/womens-health/clinical-guidance/amniocentesis-and-chorionic-villus-sampling-green-top-8].

2. Royal College of Obstetricians and Gynaecologists. *Use of Anti-D Immunoglobulin for Rh Prophylaxis*. Green-top Guideline No. 22. London: RCOG; 2002 [www.rcog.org.uk/womens-health/clinical-guidance/use-anti-d-immunoglobulin-rh-prophylaxis-green-top-22].

3. Tabor A, Philip J, Madsen M, Bang J, Obel EB, Norgaard-Pedersen B. Randomised controlled trial of genetic amniocentesis in 4606 low-risk women. *Lancet* 1986;i:1287–93.

4. Eddleman K, Malone F, Sullivan L, Dukes K, Berkowitz RL, Kharbutli Y, et al. Pregnancy loss rates after midtrimester amniocentesis. *Obstet Gynecol* 2006;108:1067-1072.

5. Mujezinovic F, Alfirevic Z. Procedure-related complications of amniocentesis and chorionic villus sampling: a systematic review. *Obstet Gynecol* 2007;110:687–94.

6. Odibo A, Gray D, Dicke J, Stamilio D, Macones G, Crane J. Revisiting the fetal loss rate after second-trimester genetic amniocentesis: a single center's 16-year experience. *Obstet Gynecol* 2008;111:589–95.

7. Canadian Early and Mid-trimester Amniocentesis Trial (CEMAT) Group. Randomised trial to assess safety and fetal outcome of early and midtrimester amniocentesis. *Lancet* 1998;351:242–7.

8. Alfirevic Z, Mujezinovic F, Sundberg K. Amniocentesis and chorionic villus sampling for prenatal diagnosis. *Cochrane Database Syst Rev* 2008;(4).

9. Tietung Hospital of Ansham Iron and Steel Company. Fetal sex prediction by sex chromatin of chorionic villi cells during early pregnancy. *Chinese Med J* 1975;2:118–25.

10. Daffos F, Capella-Pavlovsky M, Forestier F. A new procedure for fetal blood sampling in utero: preliminary results of fifty-three cases. *Am J Obstet Gynecol* 1983;146:985–7.

11. Tongsong T, Wanapirak C, Kunavikatikul C, Sirirchotiyakul S, Piyamongkol W, Chanprapaph P. Fetal loss rate associated with cordocentesis at mid-gestation. *Am J Obstet Gynecol* 2001;184:710–23.

12. American College of Obstetricians and Gynecologists. Invasive prenatal testing for aneuploidy. ACOG Practice Bulletin No. 88. *Obstet Gynecol* 2007;110:1459–67.

13. Lo YMD, Corbetta N, Chamberlain PF, Rai V, Sargent IL, Redman CW, et al. Presence of fetal DNA in maternal plasma and serum. *Lancet* 1997:350;485–7.

3 The routine anomaly scan

Introduction

Since the inception of ultrasound into routine antenatal care, its role has diversified from simply confirming fetal viability and establishing gestational age to assessment of the fetus *in utero*. With improved resolution, fetal organs can be visualised in fine detail, allowing comprehensive evaluation of the fetal anatomy.

Structural fetal abnormalities occur in approximately 2–3% of all pregnancies. In addition, they account for almost 10% of stillbirths and 25% of all neonatal deaths. Some pregnant women are at increased risk

Table 3.1	Risk factors for congenital malformations	
Risk factor	*Abnormality*	*Risk (%)*
Family history		
Neural tube defect (NTD)	NTD	5
Congenital heart disease (CHD)	CHD	5
Cleft lip/palate in parent	Cleft lip/palate	4
Medication		
Anticonvulsants (monotherapy)	NTD, CHD, cleft lip/palate	3–6
Warfarin	Bone and facial	25
Lithium	Ebstein's anomaly	7
Retinoic acid	Craniofacial, central nervous system (CNS)	23–28
Angiotensin-converting enzyme (ACE) inhibitors	CHD, CNS, renal	7
Maternal medical disease		
Insulin-dependent diabetes	CHD, NTD	9
Phenylketonuria	CHD, CNS	2–17
Maternal infection (first trimester)		
Rubella	Cataract, deafness,	80
Cytomegalovirus	CNS, deafness, fetal growth restriction	10–25
Other		
Multiple pregnancy	CHD, CNS	2–3

of structural fetal abnormalities (Table 3.1). These women can be selected for detailed ultrasound examination of the fetus and congenital abnormalities identified or excluded. Unfortunately, the majority of fetal abnormalities occur in women with no underlying or identifiable risk factors. To detect these abnormalities, a screening test within the general obstetric population is required.

By definition, a screening test should identify specific conditions within apparently healthy individuals, with a view to reducing the morbidity and mortality associated with the conditions in question. The test needs to be safe, easy to perform, reliable and have auditable standards. Routine mid-trimester ultrasound examination of all pregnant women was introduced to screen for structural fetal abnormalities in the 'normal' or 'low-risk' obstetric population. This chapter outlines the current recommendations for mid-trimester scanning, evaluates the effectiveness of the test and looks at future developments that aim to address some of the current difficulties with screening for structural fetal abnormality.

Second-trimester anomaly scans

The Royal College of Obstetricians and Gynaecologists published guidelines for the 20-week anomaly scan in 2000.[1] Subsequently, in 2008, the National Institute for Health and Clinical Excellence advised that all pregnant women should be offered this test as part of routine antenatal care (Box 3.1).[2] Despite these recommendations, the provision of routine anomaly scans, the standards applied and the detection rates attained varied considerably throughout the country. In an effort to remove these disparities and to standardise the ultrasound screening services available, the UK National Screening Committee has published recommendations of the fetal anomaly ultrasound screening service to be provided for all pregnant women in England.[3]

Routine second-trimester anomaly scans are currently performed between 18^{+0} and 20^{+6} weeks of gestation. While women are generally keen to have their scan as soon as possible, there is clear evidence that delaying the routine anomaly scan until around 20 weeks of gestation increases the likelihood of obtaining satisfactory images, achieving a complete examination with one visit and identifying fetal problems.

Minimum standards for the 20-week anomaly scan

Fetal anatomy should be examined using standard views. To confirm normality, certain key aspects ought to be identified within each view obtained. Table 3.2 and Figure 3.1a–i outline and illustrate each of these sections and their essential components. The new guidelines published for England have emphasised that examination of the outflow tracts of

BOX 3.1   EXTRACT FROM THE NCC-WCH RECOMMENDATIONS ON SCREENING FOR FETAL ANOMALIES[2]

Ultrasound screening for fetal anomalies should be routinely offered, normally between 18 weeks 0 days and 20 weeks 6 days.

At the first contact with a healthcare professional, women should be given information about the purpose and implications of the anomaly scan to enable them to make an informed choice as to whether or not to have the scan. The purpose of the scan is to identify fetal anomalies and allow:

- reproductive choice (termination of pregnancy)
- parents to prepare (for any treatment/disability/palliative care/termination of pregnancy)
- managed birth in a specialist centre
- intrauterine therapy.

Women should be informed of the limitations of routine ultrasound screening and that detection rates vary by the type of fetal anomaly, the woman's body mass index and the position of the unborn baby at the time of the scan.

If an anomaly is detected during the anomaly scan pregnant women should be informed of the findings to enable them to make an informed choice as to whether they wish to continue with the pregnancy or have a termination of pregnancy.

Fetal echocardiography involving the four chamber view of the fetal heart and outflow tracts is recommended as part of the routine anomaly scan.

Routine screening for cardiac anomalies using nuchal translucency is not recommended.

When routine ultrasound screening is performed to detect neural tube defects, alphafetoprotein testing is not required.

Participation in regional congenital anomaly registers and/or UK National Screening Committee approved audit systems is strongly recommended to facilitate the audit of detection rates.

the heart and of the face and lips should be included in every anomaly scan. While it is likely that this will improve the overall detection rate of fetal abnormalities, identifying these features requires supplementary training, adds extra time to the ultrasound examination and increases the recall rate, as both facial and cardiac views require the fetus to be in an optimal position.

Each unit must ensure that local department protocols reflect the recommendations outlined in the NHS Fetal Anomaly Screening Programme (NHS FASP). In addition, the guidelines have highlighted the minimum

Table 3.2   Checklist for a second-trimester routine anomaly scan

Views examined	Features to be identified
Head	Cavum septum pellucidum Cerebellum × 2 lobes and vermis Posterior fossa < 6 mm Lateral ventricles: posterior horn < 10 mm Nuchal fold
Face	Normal facial profile 2 orbits Lips and nostrils
Spine	Longitudinal and transverse sections of vertebrae, confirming integrity of skin cover
Abdomen at level of stomach	Shape and contents of abdomen Stomach on left side of abdomen Clear demarcation between abdomen and thorax
Cord insertion	Intact abdominal wall 3 vessels in cord
Abdomen at level of kidneys	Both kidneys identified Renal pelvis < 5 mm Bladder
4-chamber view of heart	Correctly orientated Appropriate size 4 chambers Independent valves Intact septum Aorta and pulmonary artery
Arms	Three bones in each arm Hand × 2 Digits on each hand not counted
Legs	Three bones in each leg Foot × 2 Toes on each foot not counted

standards expected for image storage and documentation during an anomaly scan (page 74 of NHS FASP document).[3]

Detection rates

Given the wide variation in the standards and practice for routine anomaly scanning to date, it is not surprising that the detection rates for fetal abnormality before 24 weeks of gestation have also varied considerably. The majority of studies performed in the late 1990s consistently

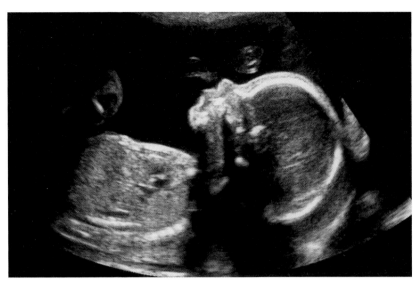

Figure 3.1a A longitudinal section through the fetus demonstrating a normal facial profile

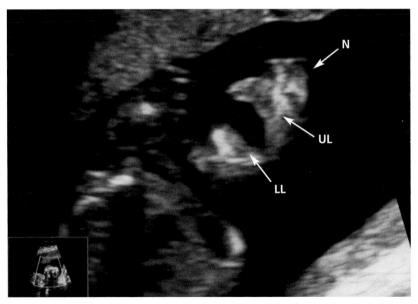

Figure 3.1b A frontal image of the face illustrating the fetal nose (N), upper lip (UL) and lower lip (LL)

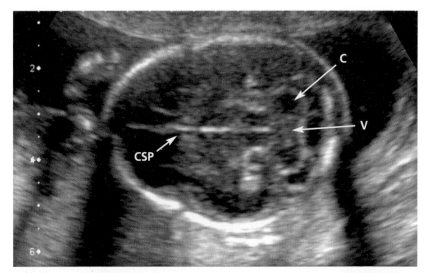

Figure 3.1c A transverse section of a normal oval-shaped fetal head. (C) cerebellum (V) vermis of cerebellum (CSP) cavum septum pellucidum

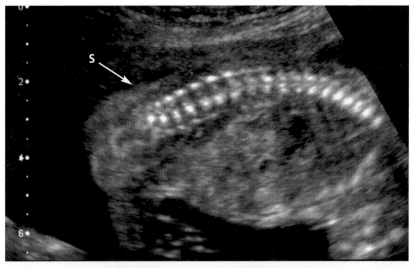

Figure 3.1d The fetal spine in longitudinal section, with the two vertebral columns merging at the fetal coccyx and a complete layer of skin (S) seen to overlie the bones throughout

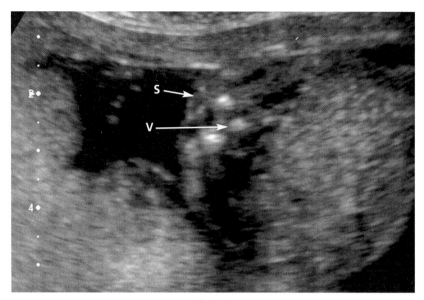

Figure 3.1e A transverse section of the fetal spine with the three points of the vertebral bone (V) and an intact skin layer (S)

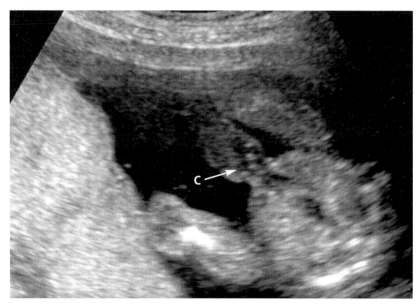

Figure 3.1f A transverse section of the fetal abdomen at the level of the cord insertion (CI)

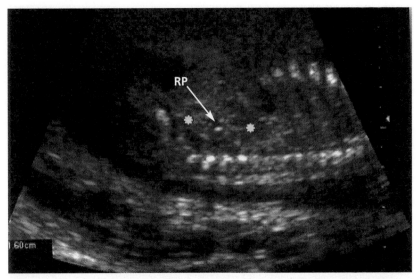

Figure 3.1g The fetal kidney in long section – with the small renal pelvis (RP) identified

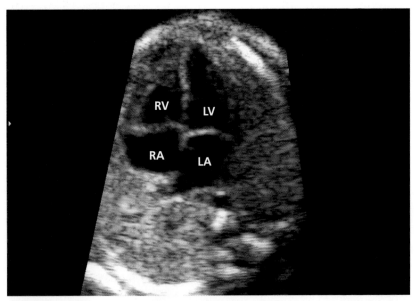

Figure 3.1h A transverse section of the fetal chest with a normal 4 chamber view of the fetal heart (RV) right ventricle (LV) left ventricle (RA) right atrium (LA) left atrium

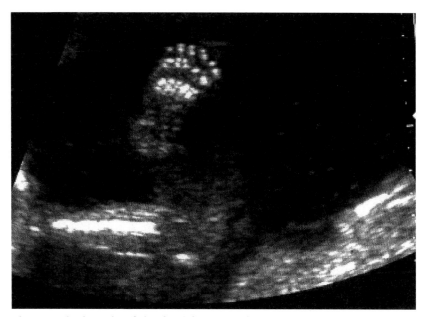

Figure 3.1i The sole of the fetal foot with five digits seen

demonstrated that 50–70% of major structural abnormalities were detected, even in low-risk populations. Table 3.3 lists a sample of these studies and illustrates the wide diversity of detection rates for specific malformations within each study. The detection of congenital heart disease (CHD) has been consistently low. While these studies offer some guidance on 'expected' detection rates, they should be interpreted with caution. The majority are multicentre studies conducted by multiprofessional groups over a lengthy time period. In more recent years, there have been significant improvements in staff practice, training, department protocols and the equipment used. Given the spectrum of variables within each study, the results should only suggest a minimum standard that should be achieved in current practice and offer some benchmark by which current practice within each unit can be assessed. The NHS FASP has listed 11 fetal abnormalities which can be identified during a routine anomaly scan and the limited detection rates that can be expected in a national screening programme (Table 3.4).

The recent epidemic of maternal obesity has proved a major challenge to all sonographers. The resolution achieved by even the best of machinery is diminished in the presence of excessive adipose tissue and the likelihood of detecting fetal problems is therefore reduced. It is well documented that among women with diabetes, fewer fetal abnormalities are detected in those with a large body mass index (BMI).[4] The most

Table 3.3 Antenatal detection of selected congenital abnormalities during a routine anomaly scan

	SWEDEN (1999)[14] (n/N)	(%)	UK[a,b] (1998)[15] (%)	GREECE (1999)[16] (n/N)	(%)	EUROPE[b] (1999)[17] (n/N)	(%)	SWEDEN[b] (2006)[13] (n/N)	(%)
Central nervous system									
Anencephaly	3/3	100	98	27/29	93	156/157	100	6/6	100
Spina bifida	3/4	75				146/181	81	8/12	66
Congenital heart disease									
Major	0/35	0	38	14/31	45	142/366	39	8/52	15
Minor	0/35	0				122/387	31		
Gastrointestinal tract									
Anterior abdominal wall defects	2/2	100	90	23/27	85			4/6	67
Renal									
Agenesis	3/6	50	82	24/28	86	36/43	84	2/2	100
Cystic change	1/3	33				64/70	91	9/11	82
Hydronephrosis	2/9	22				508/544	93	13/14	93
Skeletal									
Major	4/6	67	85	22/26	85	257/349	74	9/18	50

[a] Multicentre studies; [b] Malformations grouped and reported by systems

Table 3.4	The 11 auditable conditions and detection rates (reproduced with permission from NHS FASP)

Condition	Detection rate (%)
Anencephaly	98
Open spina bifida	90
Cleft lip	75
Diaphragmatic hernia	60
Gastroschisis	98
Exomphalos	80
Serious cardiac abnormalities	50
Bilateral renal agenesis	84
Skeletal dysplasias	60
Trisomy 18 (Edwards syndrome)	96
Trisomy 13 (Patau syndrome)	95

skilled operators with optimal modern machinery are likely to find this an increasing burden that may well adversely influence detection rates of fetal abnormality in the future.

Despite detailed protocols with expert sonographers using good-quality machinery, some fetal abnormalities may just not be evident at 18–20 weeks of gestation and so cannot be identified at the routine anomaly scan.

Problems associated with routine anomaly scans

SOFT MARKERS

During a routine anomaly scan, minor sonographic abnormalities or 'soft markers' may be identified. These are ultrasound features that are associated with but not diagnostic of fetal problems such as aneuploidy.

Nuchal fold

The nuchal thickness can be measured on a transverse section of the head, at the level of the cerebellum that includes the posterior fossa. Normal nuchal measurements in the second trimester should be 5 mm or less. Measurements that are 6 mm or above occur in less than 1% of the population and are associated with increased risk of trisomy. An increased nuchal fold measurement at 15–20 weeks of gestation is estimated to increase the existing risk of trisomy 21 ten-fold.

Choroid plexus cysts

Choroid plexus cysts are anechoic (fluid-filled) areas of variable size, within the substance of the choroid plexus. They are seen in approximately

1% of pregnancies at 18–22 weeks of gestation and the majority regress by the end of the second trimester. The size, number, laterality and persistence or regression of choroid plexus cysts does not correlate with fetal outcome. An isolated cyst does not increase the risk of trisomy 21. It does, however, appear to increase the risk of trisomy 18 for women over the age of 36 years and those with a screen result of less than one in 3000 pregnancies, increasing their risk to within the cut-off of serum screening.[5,6]

Echogenic bowel
Fetal echogenic bowel is found in approximately 0.5–1.0% of second-trimester scans and is classified as bowel with the same echogenicity as the surrounding bones of the iliac crest. Echogenic bowel may be a normal finding but is also associated with fetal growth restriction, cystic fibrosis, placental insufficiency and aneuploidy. In the largest follow-up studies of fetal echogenic bowel, chromosome abnormalities were found in 3.5–7.0% of cases (other reviews estimating the relative risk of trisomy 21 being 5.5 times the underlying background risk), cystic fibrosis was present in 3% of cases, congenital infection in 3% and fetal growth restriction in 4%. Having excluded these problems, the vast majority of babies were normal and subsequently had no long-term problems.

Renal pelvis dilatation
The renal pelvis is measured in an anteroposterior diameter, on a transverse view of the kidneys. If the diameter exceeds a cut-off level, usually 5 mm, a diagnosis of renal pelvis dilatation or pyelectasis is made. In low-risk populations, the incidence of renal pelvis dilatation is less than 2%. It is frequently a normal variation but is also associated with trisomies and neonatal renal problems such as reflux. While up to 25% of trisomic fetuses have evidence of renal pelvis dilatation, the false-positive rate is high. It is estimated that renal pelvis dilatation has a very small impact on the underlying background risk of trisomy, particularly trisomy 21 with an increased risk of only 1.5. Therefore, in the absence of either additional abnormal scan findings or abnormal screening results, most accept that the risk of trisomy is low and invasive testing is not indicated for isolated renal pelvis dilatation.

In the absence of additional markers, a follow-up scan should be organised in the third trimester to assess liquor volume and the degree of renal pelvis dilatation. Even if renal pelvis dilatation appears to have 'resolved' in the third trimester, some babies will still have underlying urinary tract problems. Therefore, all neonates with a mid-trimester diagnosis of renal pelvis dilatation should have postnatal assessment of the urinary tract to exclude underlying problems such as reflux.[7] The neonatal management of these cases varies among paediatric departments. Local protocols should guide clinicians as to the use of antibiotics in the neonatal period, the initial investigation of choice and the timing of any such investigations.

Ventriculomegaly

The lateral ventricles of the brain normally measure less than 10 mm in anteroposterior diameter. In fetuses with an anteroposterior diameter greater than 10 mm there is an increased risk of trisomy. Ventriculomegaly can also be a marker for additional structural abnormalities of the brain and congenital infection. In spite of all these associations, it is recognised that the majority of babies with mild ventriculomegaly (10–15 mm) will have a normal outcome.

Two-vessel cord

A single umbilical artery is often found in pregnancies that have either chromosome or structural abnormalities or both. However, it is usually associated with other abnormalities and, as an isolated finding, it is not therefore used to adjust the risk of trisomy 21. The incidence of single umbilical artery in normal pregnancies varies from 0.5% to 1.5% depending on the method of ascertainment used.

Echogenic foci in the heart

Echogenic areas, 'golf balls', may be seen in up to 10% of normal pregnancies and occur more frequently in pregnancies of Asian mothers. The foci are associated with the papillary muscles in the ventricle and move with the related valves throughout the cardiac cycle. They are present owing to mineralisation of the papillary muscles and are more commonly seen within the left ventricle. It is generally accepted that if echogenic foci are the only soft marker present, the risk of trisomy is not increased in low-risk populations.

Summary of soft markers

Second-trimester soft markers were all initially described and used to refine the risk of trisomy in women in high-risk groups. With the introduction of routine second-trimester anomaly scanning, the low-risk population was subjected to the same level of ultrasound assessment. This, coupled with apprehension of the threat of litigation, encouraged widespread disclosure of all scan findings in many units, however minor they appeared or however low the association with fetal trisomy.

The majority of women who attend for second-trimester anomaly scans have had some form of screening, either first-trimester nuchal screening or second-trimester biochemical screening. These women are not screened 'positive' until they reach a threshold, usually a risk greater than one in 250. For the vast majority of women with a low-risk screening result, the presence of a single soft marker will not adjust this result into the 'screen positive' group. Some units have therefore opted either to ignore soft markers completely or to only advise mothers of the increased risk of trisomy if two or more soft markers were identified during the anomaly scan.

To standardise the use of soft markers identified during an anomaly scan, the NHS FASP has included guidance on this issue. It is recommended that the term 'Down's soft marker' should no longer be used. The ultrasound findings of choroid plexus cysts, a dilated cistern magna, echogenic foci in the heart and a two-vessel cord should no longer initiate a referral for aneuploidy counselling. However, increased nuchal translucency greater than 6 mm, dilated renal pelvis (greater than 7 mm) ventriculomegaly (greater than 10 mm) and echogenic bowel (with the same density as bone), all associated with multiple pathologies in addition to aneuploidy, should be referred for further assessment and, if indicated, additional testing.

FALSE POSITIVE SCAN FINDINGS

Irregularities seen during the anomaly ultrasound examination may be real and even persistent over several scans but following delivery no abnormality can be found in the neonate and repeated investigations prove normal. Common examples of these 'irregularities' are cystic areas within the fetal abdomen, chest and pelvis, dilated loops of bowel, abnormalities in the brain tissue and echogenic areas within the chest or abdomen. Clearly, at the time of fetal ultrasound, parents need to be informed of the findings and of the possible diagnosis that they represent. For many parents, there ensues a period of anxious waiting until delivery when more formal investigations can establish the veracity of the antenatal findings.

More commonly, during a routine anomaly scan, the sonographer may be unable, for a variety of reasons, to confirm that an organ is normal. Once more, a period of anxiety ensues for parents while a second opinion is organised and the findings are either confirmed or refuted. There are no good national studies looking at the number of scans requiring a second opinion, nor the mean time that parents have to wait for clarity.

The psychological impact of these events on parents is often poorly appreciated. It is important that adequate support systems exist within each department to help parents cope with the weeks of uncertainty until such time as a clear diagnosis is reached.

FALSE-NEGATIVE SCAN FINDINGS

While some parents face weeks of uncertainty, others may have been reassured by an apparently normal scan, only to be shocked by the diagnosis of a fetal abnormality, either at a later stage in the pregnancy or following delivery. There are several reasons why this may occur. The mandatory views for a routine 20-week anomaly scan are determined by individual departments. Abnormalities may therefore be 'missed' because they do not fall into the list of structures to be evaluated. Even with the most stringent protocols in place, some abnormalities cannot be detected, as they are very difficult to detect at 20 weeks or they may not present until a later stage in pregnancy. For example, the diagnostic features of critical aortic stenosis and duodenal atresia may not be evident in the second-trimester fetus. Likewise, the stomach may appear in an appropriate position at 18 weeks of gestation but may be clearly seen within the chest cavity at 26 weeks owing to a diaphragmatic hernia. The other abnormalities commonly 'missed' for this reason are hydrocephalus, microcephaly, renal abnormalities, cleft palate, ovarian cysts and other types of CHD. In addition, despite repeated ultrasound scans, limitations in imaging, particularly in women who are obese, may never be overcome and abnormalities may be missed. Finally, as the RADIUS study demonstrated, abnormalities may not be recognised because of inadequately trained personnel or inappropriate machinery being used for the examination.[8] For this reason the Royal College of Obstetricians and Gynaecologists and the NHS FASP have detailed the competency that is expected of personnel undertaking routine anomaly scans.[1,3,9]

For the future

THE FIRST-TRIMESTER ANOMALY SCAN

With improvements in ultrasound imaging, it is possible to examine the first-trimester fetus for structural abnormalities. Initial studies, primarily in tertiary centres, have shown promising results. Using a combination of transabdominal and transvaginal examinations, 70% of significant abnormalities were identified at 12–14 weeks of gestation.[10] However, subsequent studies have failed to replicate this success on a consistent basis. While almost all cases of anencephaly were diagnosed by 14 weeks, the overall detection rate for all other malformations at a 12–14 week examination has ranged from 20% to 60%.[11–13] As with the second-trimester scan, there are multiple reasons for this diversity, including quality of machinery, staff experience, fetal position and the delayed presentation of some abnormalities. The use of transvaginal scans as a first-line approach in the first trimester does not appear to improve the detection rates achieved, since there is a limited range of movement available with the probe and adequate examination depends largely on appropriate fetal orientation and movement at the time of scanning.

Fetal anatomy changes significantly between the first and second

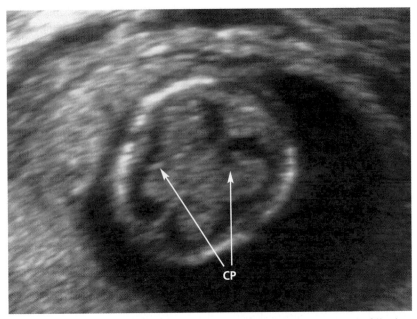

Figure 3.2 The first trimester fetal choroid plexus (CP) completely fills the lateral ventricles and occupies most of the hemisphere

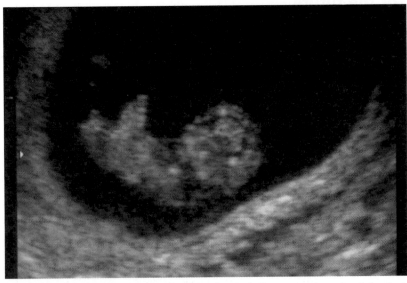

Figure 3.3 A transverse section of the fetal abdomen with a physiological herniation of the fetal gut

trimesters. The sonographer must appreciate the dynamic changes that occur to ensure that fetal malformations are not over or misdiagnosed. The choroid plexus is relatively large and fills the lateral ventricle, which in turn occupies most of the cranial hemisphere (Figure 3.2). By the second trimester, the relative size of the ventricle and choroid plexus diminishes and, where the ventricular measurements remain large, this is an abnormal finding. Intra-abdominal bowel can clearly be seen outside the abdomen until at least 11–12 weeks of gestation before returning to the abdominal cavity. It is only where this physiological herniation (Figure 3.3) does not correct, by a fetal crown–rump length of 68 mm, that gastroschisis should be diagnosed. In addition, the fetal bowel may protrude into the base of the umbilical cord in the 12–14 week period but this may be a normal 'variation' and should not be presumed to be exomphalos. The fetal kidneys and bladder may be difficult to visualise at around 12 weeks of gestation but this does not mean there is absence of the fetal kidneys.

With continued improvements in ultrasound technology, increasing sonographer experience and the drive towards first-trimester aneuploidy screening, it is likely that a greater number of fetal abnormalities will be identified in the first trimester.

THREE- AND FOUR-DIMENSIONAL ULTRASOUND

Three-dimensional (3-D)and real-time (four-dimensional, 4-D) ultrasound imaging facilities are now available on most mid-range ultrasound machines. To date, 3-D imaging has primarily been used to augment two-dimensional (2-D) scanning. There is clear evidence that it helps to define or verify the presence of facial or surface-based abnormalities such as exophthalmia and facial clefting.

Each 3-D image acquired contains a large series of 2-D image planes. These are digitally stored and can be evaluated at a later time. Using computer software, these fetal planes can be viewed in sequence, remote from the mother, in a similar manner to magnetic resonance imaging. This raises many possibilities for routine anomaly scanning in the future; improved efficiency of examination within departments, fewer incomplete examinations, standardisation of the structures examined and potentially improved detection of fetal abnormalities.

WHAT DO PARENTS EXPECT?

Few women refuse the option of an 18–20 week ultrasound scan. It is perceived to be a safe investigation with no risk to the pregnancy. Most parents attend the assessment, expecting to be reassured about the wellbeing of their pregnancy, but few appreciate either the limitations or the function of an anomaly scan. While the diagnosis of an adverse outcome or an abnormal finding generates a 'shock' response, studies consistently suggest that women wish to be informed of fetal abnormalities and continue to seek ultrasound screening in further pregnancies. They perceive the positive effects of seeing the fetus and being reassured to outweigh the small possibility of a fetal abnormality being identified.

In those pregnancies where a problem is identified, early diagnosis offers time for adequate counselling and, where indicated, referral to other centres for additional tests, *in utero* therapy or planned delivery. When lethal or severe abnormalities are identified, the early diagnosis of fetal abnormality allows parents choice and the option of termination of the pregnancy. Those who are initially reassured but who later during the pregnancy or following delivery are informed of a fetal abnormality, find the process more difficult to deal with.

Summary

Owing to the range of fetal abnormalities and the spectrum of presentation, a single ultrasound examination in either the first or second trimester will never detect all fetal malformations. Given current economic, equipment and staffing constraints, the second-trimester scan at 20 weeks of gestation is the single most useful scan for detecting fetal abnormality. Those performing this critical examination must be adequately trained to ensure the optimal number of fetal abnormalities is detected. Robust data collection of pregnancy outcomes within each unit is essential to verify that these standards are achieved and maintained in the long term. While improved imaging, first-trimester 3-D and 4-D scans may increase the detection rates of fetal anomalies, fetal abnormality is but one cause of fetal morbidity and mortality and no pregnancy can be guaranteed a completely 'normal' outcome.

References

1. Royal College of Obstetricians and Gynaecologists. *Routine Ultrasound Screening in Pregnancy: Protocol, Standards and Training. Supplement to Ultrasound Screening for Fetal Abnormalities: Report of the RCOG Working Party*. London: RCOG; 2000 [www.rcog.org.uk/womens-health/clinical-guidance/ultrasound-screening].

2. National Collaborating Centre for Women's and Children's Health. *Antenatal Care: Routine Care for the Healthy Pregnant Women*. 2nd ed. London: RCOG Press; 2008 [http://guidance.nice.org.uk/CG62]. p. 134–52.

3. NHS Fetal Anomaly Screening Programme. The 18+0 to 20+6 weeks fetal anomaly scan: your online resource. [www.fetalanomalyscreening.nhs.uk].

4. Wong SF, Chan FY, Cincotta RB, Oats JJ, McIntyre HD. Routine ultrasound screening in diabetic pregnancies. *Ultrasound Obstet Gynecol* 2002;19:171–6.

5. Chitty LS, Chudleigh P, Wright E, Campbell S, Pembrey M. The significance of choroid plexus cysts in an unselected population: results of a multicentre study. *Ultrasound Obstet Gynecol* 1998;12:391–7.

6. Yoder P, Sabbagha R, Gross S, Zelop C. The second trimester fetus with isolated choroid plexus cysts: a meta-analysis of risk of trisomies 18 and 21. *Obstet Gynecol* 1999;93:869–72.

7. Duncan KA. Antenatal renal pelvic dilatation; the long -term outlook. *Clin Radiol* 2007;62:134–9.

8. Ewigman BG, Crane JP, Frigoletto FD, LeFevre ML, Bain RP, McNellis D; RADIUS Study Group. Effect of prenatal ultrasound screening on perinatal outcome. *N Engl J Med* 1993;329:821–7.

9. Royal College of Obstetricians and Gynaecologists. *Ultrasound Screening for Fetal Abnormalities: Report of the RCOG Working Party*. London: RCOG; 1997.

10. Braithwaite JM, Armstrong MA, Economides DL. The assessment of fetal anatomy at 12–13 weeks using transabdominal and transvaginal sonography. *Br J Obstet Gynaecol* 1996;103:82–5.

11. Economides D, Braithwaite JM. First trimester sonographic diagnosis of fetal structural abnormalities in a low risk population *Br J Obstet Gynaecol* 1998;105;53–7.

12. Carvalho MH, Brizot ML, Lopes LM, Chiba CH, Miyadahira S Zugaib M. Detection of fetal structural abnormalities at the 11–14 weeks scan. *Prenat Diagn* 2002;22:1–4.

13. Svaltvedt S, Almstrom H, Kublickas M, Valentin L, Grunewald C. Detection of malformations in chromosomally normal fetuses by routine ultrasound at 12 or 18 weeks of gestation: a randomised controlled trial in 39 572 pregnancies. *BJOG* 2006;113:664–74.

14. Eurenius K, Axelsson O, Cnattingius S, Eriksson L, Norsted T. Second trimester ultrasound screening performed by midwives; sensitivity for detection of fetal abnormalities. *Acta Obstet Gynecol Scand* 1999;78:98–104.

15. Boyd PA, Chamberlain P, Hicks NR. 6-year experience of prenatal diagnosis in an unselected population in Oxford, UK. *Lancet* 1998;352:577–81.

16. Stefos T, Plachouras N, Sotiriadis A, Papadimitriou D, Almoussa N, Navrozoglou I, *et al*. Routine obstetrical ultrasound at 18–22 weeks: our experience on 7,236 fetuses. *J Matern Fetal Med* 1999;8:64–9.

17. Grandjean H, Larroque D, Levi S. The performance of routine ultrasonographic screening of pregnancies in the Eurofetus Study. *Am J Obstet Gynecol* 1999;181:446–54.

4 Fetal structural abnormalities

Introduction

Approximately 3% of pregnancies are affected by a single major structural malformation. The frequency of structural anomaly is higher at conception but declines owing to the natural attrition rate associated with abnormal fetuses. Congenital malformation has multiple aetiologies, as illustrated in Table 4.1. As discussed in Chapter 3, antenatal diagnosis of fetal anomaly may have important implications for the subsequent management of the pregnancy. A comprehensive discussion of structural abnormalities is beyond the scope of this chapter, which should be viewed as an introduction to the subject.

Central nervous system

Neural tube defects comprise anencephaly (40%), spina bifida (55%) and encephalocele (5%). Risk factors for these conditions are shown in Table 4.2. There is geographical variation in the frequency of neural tube defects, the west of Scotland and Ireland having the highest incidence in Great Britain. The birth incidence of these conditions has fallen, with an estimated 2/1000 cases in the west of Scotland. The reason for this decline in birth frequency is unknown and is not simply because of the option of termination of an affected pregnancy.

Table 4.1   Aetiology of congenital malformation

Aetiology	Type (%)
Idiopathic	60.0
Multifactorial	20.0
Single gene disorder	7.5
Chromosomal	6.0
Maternal illness	3.0
Congenital infection	2.0
Drugs, X-ray, alcohol	1.5

Table 4.2   Risk factors for neural tube defects

Factor	Example
Elevated maternal serum alphafetoprotein	
Family history	Risk 1/25 if one affected parent or sibling Risk 1/10 if two affected siblings
Maternal disorder	Diabetes mellitus, epilepsy
Drugs	Sodium valproate, phenytoin, carbamazepine
Chromosomal abnormalities	Trisomy 18, trisomy 13
Single gene mutations	Meckel–Gruber syndrome (autosomal recessive)

Screening programmes for neural tube defects were introduced in the 1970s. They rely on estimation of maternal serum alphafetoprotein (AFP) concentrations and results are expressed as multiples of the median (MoM). Individual screening programmes employ a cut-off point that maximises detection of affected pregnancies while maintaining an acceptable false-positive rate. Screening is performed between 15 and 21 weeks of gestation, the optimum time being 16–18 weeks, and in the west of Scotland an AFP level of 2 MoM or greater will detect 100% of cases of anencephaly and 80% of cases of open spina bifida. The diagnostic test following a positive screening test result for neural tube defects is ultrasound, which will detect 100% of cases of anencephaly and 98% of cases of open spina bifida.

ANENCEPHALY

In anencephaly, there is absence of the cerebral hemispheres and most of the cranial vault. This results in prominent orbits and the typical 'frog-like' appearance on transabdominal ultrasound (Figure 4.1). It is a lethal condition, occurring more commonly in female fetuses.

SPINA BIFIDA

Spina bifida results from the failure of closure of the neural groove, a process that is normally complete by 28 days post-conception. The lesion may be open (Figure 4.2) or closed, the latter having a skin covering. Closed lesions are usually small, AFP levels are not increased and antenatal detection by ultrasound is frequently not possible. In open lesions, the bony spine and overlying skin are disrupted and a bulging

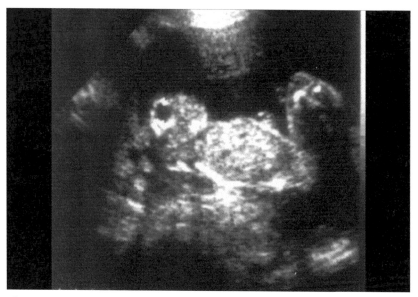

Figure 4.1 Anencephaly: the cranial vault is absent and the orbits are prominent producing the characteristic 'frog-like' appearance

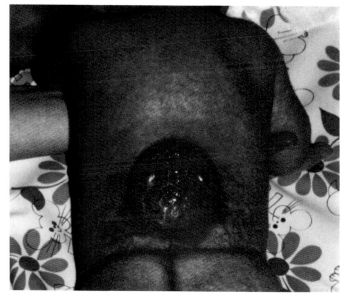

Figure 4.2 Open spina bifida

meningeal membrane is apparent. If neural tissue is present within the sac, it is termed a myelomeningocele. The lumbosacral area is most commonly affected. The 'lemon' and 'banana' signs describe the cranial features seen on ultrasound that are associated with spina bifida. The 'lemon' sign refers to the shape of the head as a result of scalloping of the frontal bones (Figure 4.3). The Arnold–Chiari malformation (type II) is defined as descent of the cerebellum, pons and medulla through the foramen magnum, leading to obliteration of the cisterna magna (Figure 4.4). The resulting 'banana' shape of the cerebellum is pathognomonic for spina bifida. The degree of handicap can be difficult to predict in the antenatal period. The extent of physical handicap depends in part on the site and size of the lesion and there may be gross paralysis of the lower limbs with bladder and bowel dysfunction. Intelligence can be normal but it is impossible to predict this *in utero*. Owing to the potential for a poor prognosis, termination of pregnancy is one of the options available. Those couples choosing to continue with the pregnancy should have access to multidisciplinary counselling and a unit with a neonatal surgical department.

ENCEPHALOCELE

Encephalocele accounts for approximately 5% of neural tube defects. The lesion is most commonly occipital (75%) and intracranial contents protrude through a bony defect in the skull (Figure 4.5). It is important to demonstrate a bony defect to differentiate encephalocele from other causes of soft tissue swelling, such as cystic hygroma or hydrops. Up to 15% of encephaloceles have a coexistent spina bifida lesion.

ADDITIONAL ANOMALIES

Detection of a structural abnormality on ultrasound should always lead to a thorough search for additional anomalies, since their presence can alter the diagnosis, management and implications for a future pregnancy. For example, a fetus with an isolated neural tube defect may be managed entirely differently from a fetus with a neural tube defect and an exomphalos, which could indicate trisomy 18, a generally lethal condition. Alternatively, a neural tube defect and polycystic kidneys suggest a diagnosis of Meckel–Gruber syndrome, which has a recurrence risk of one in four, in contrast to a recurrence risk of 1/25 for an isolated lesion. In the presence of multiple defects karyotyping should be offered.

Preconceptional folic acid supplementation, 0.4 mg daily, reduces the incidence of neural tube defects. Women who have had a previously affected pregnancy or who are taking anticonvulsants should take a higher daily dose (4 mg).

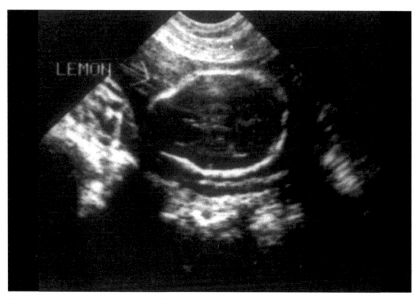

Figure 4.3 'Lemon' sign; scalloping of the frontal bones gives the skull a lemon shape

VENTRICULOMEGALY

Ventriculomegaly is described as a lateral ventricular diameter of 10–15 mm, irrespective of gestational age. In the normal fetus, the mean lateral ventricular diameter is around 7 mm and this remains stable throughout gestation. Mild bilateral ventriculomegaly affects 0.15–0.7% of pregnancies.[1] While the outcome of isolated mild bilateral ventriculomegaly is

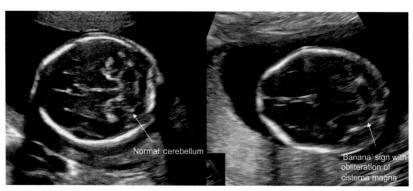

Figure 4.4 Normal cerebellum (left); 'banana'-shaped cerebellum (right), indicative of neural tube defect

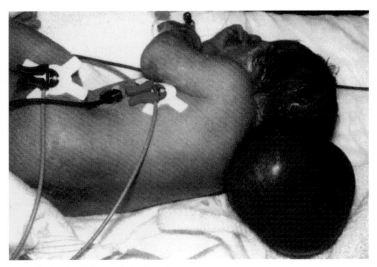

Figure 4.5 Occipital encephalocele

favourable in the majority of cases, there are some associations, which are summarised in a review of the literature presented in Table 4.3.[2]

Table 4.3	Outcome of isolated mild bilateral ventriculomegaly (data from Pilu *et al.* 1999)[2]				
Series	Aneuploidy (%)	Structural anomalies (NK) (%)	Perinatal deaths (NK) (%)	Developmental delay (NK) (%)	Abnormal outcome (total cases) (%)
Mahoney	6.7	21.4	28.6	10	46.6
Bromley	0	3.7	0	19.2	19.2
Achiron	28.6	40	0	0	57.1
Patel	2.7	16.7	5.6	17.6	32.4
Alagappan	0	18.2	0	0	18.2
Bloom	0	3.3	3.3	31	33.3
Vergani	4.2	2.2	2.2	0	8.3
Lipitz	3.6	0	0	3.8	7.4
Pilu	6.4	12	0	8	22.2
TOTAL	3.8	8.6	3.7	11.5	22.8
NK = normal karyotype					

The incidence of chromosomal abnormality is approximately 4%, most commonly trisomy 21, and karyotyping should be discussed. Some of the structural anomalies associated with ventriculomegaly may not be detected at the first scan. Serial ultrasound assessment is therefore essential and the prognosis will change if further anomalies are detected. Magnetic resonance imaging is an important adjunct to diagnosis of additional central nervous system anomalies.

An atrial width of greater than 12 mm, progressive enlargement and asymmetrical bilateral ventriculomegaly increase the risk of an unfavourable outcome.[3]

Regardless of timing of initial diagnosis, normal developmental outcome has been documented in at least 85% of cases.[4]

HYDROCEPHALUS

Hydrocephalus is an increase in the intracranial content of cerebrospinous fluid, which results in ventriculomegaly (Figure 4.6). By definition, the lateral ventricles will have a lateral atrial diameter greater than 15 mm. The mechanisms leading to hydrocephalus are:

- obstruction to flow, such as aqueductal stenosis, which may be genetic (X-linked recessive), caused by infection (cytomegalovirus, toxoplasmosis or syphilis) or by teratogens, haemorrhage, tumours or mass lesions
- impaired cerebrospinal fluid resorption
- overproduction of cerebrospinal fluid
- underdevelopment/destruction of cortical tissue.

Obstruction is the most common aetiology. Ultrasound diagnosis relies on demonstrating an increase in the size of some or all of the ventricles. The condition is referred to as isolated hydrocephalus provided that

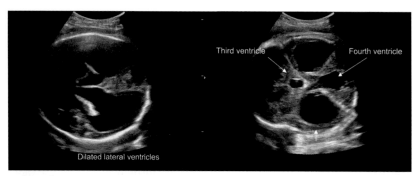

Figure 4.6 Hydrocephalus – dilated lateral ventricles (left); dilatation of entire ventricular system (right)

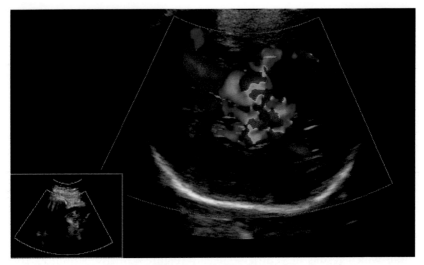

Figure 4.7 Vein of Galen aneurysm, defined by colour Doppler

there are no other structural abnormalities. However, approximately one-third of cases have additional anomalies, the most common being spina bifida, and about 10% of fetuses with hydrocephalus will have a karyotypic abnormality.

FURTHER AETIOLOGIES OF INTRACRANIAL ABNORMALITY

Abnormal intracranial anatomy should prompt consideration of other pathologies. Is there evidence of intracranial haemorrhage? If so, further assessment regarding possible neonatal alloimmune thrombocytopenia is necessary. The features may be suggestive of congenital infection, in which case screening for cytomegalovirus and toxoplasmosis is indicated, as discussed in Chapter 10. Rare anomalies, such as a vein of Galen aneurysm, can be diagnosed by application of colour Doppler (Figure 4.7), and should be suspected if there is an intracranial anomaly and evidence of cardiac failure.

Cardiovascular system

Congenital heart disease (CHD) accounts for 6–10% of neonatal deaths and 20–40% of deaths arising from congenital abnormality. The livebirth frequency of different types of CHD is shown in Table 4.4.[5] Risk factors for CHD are illustrated in Table 4.5. Detection rates for CHD depend on a number of factors. The level of cardiac scan performed is important. Solely looking at the four-chamber view will allow detection of only 40–50% of cases of CHD. Anomalies that can be detected from the four-chamber

Table 4.4 Distribution of congenital heart disease in liveborn affected infants (adapted with permission from Hoffman and Christianson 1978)[5]

Lesion	Frequency (%)
Ventricular septal defect	30.3
Pulmonary stenosis	7.4
Atrial septal defect	6.7
Aortic stenosis	5.2
Tetralogy of Fallot	5.1
Transposition of great vessels	4.7
Atrioventricular septal defect	3.2
Hypoplastic left heart syndrome	1.3
Truncus arteriosus	1.0

Table 4.5 Risk factors for congenital heart disease

Type of risk	Factor
Familial	One affected sibling recurrence risk 2–5% Two affected siblings 10–15%
Maternal:	
Medical conditions	Diabetes, systemic lupus erythematosus, phenylketonuria
Drugs	Anticonvulsants, lithium, alcohol, amphetamines, heroin, cocaine, thalidomide
Infections	Rubella, toxoplasmosis, cytomegalovirus
Fetal:	
Extracardiac anomalies	Hydrocephalus, Dandy-Walker malformation, oesophageal atresia, exomphalos, diaphragmatic hernia, renal agenesis, single umbilical artery
Non-immune hydrops	
Fetal arrhythmias	
Symmetrical FGR	
Polyhydramnios	
Chromosomal abnormalities	Trisomy 21, trisomy 18, trisomy 13, 45X

FGR = fetal growth restriction

BOX 4.1 CARDIAC ANOMALIES DETECTED ACCORDING TO TYPE OF ULTRASOUND EXAMINATION

Four-chamber view

- Atrioventricular septal defect
- Mitral atresia
- Tricuspid atresia
- Pulmonary atresia with intact septum
- Large ventricular septal defect
- Severe coarctation of the aorta
- Interrupted aortic arch
- Ebstein's anomaly
- Hypoplastic left heart syndrome

Four-chamber view + outflow tracts

- Tetralogy of Fallot
- Transposition of great arteries
- Pulmonary atresia with ventricular septal defect
- Double outlet right ventricle
- Truncus arteriosus communis

view alone are detailed in Box 4.1. Addition of the outflow tracts improves detection rates by 25–30% and ensures that all critical cases of CHD (such as transposition of the great vessels) are included.[4,6] Extended fetal echocardiography with colour flow mapping can result in detection rates of 88%.[7] There is wide variation in the detection rates reported in the literature, reflecting the level of experience and training of the operators. The detection rates quoted above will not be achieved without appropriate training and audit of practice. Early fetal echocardiography, at 14 weeks of gestation, is offered by some centres to women in high-risk groups.[8] This has the advantage of providing early information but it must be followed by a further scan at 20–22 weeks of gestation, since 20% of cases of CHD will not be detectable until that time. Irrespective of the type and timing of the scan and experience of the sonographer, some defects cannot be detected antenatally. These include secundum atrial septal defects, mild forms of aortic stenosis, pulmonary stenosis and coarctation of the aorta, and small ventricular septal defects. Women must be counselled to this effect.

EXTRACARDIAC ANOMALIES

Up to 44% of congenital heart lesions are associated with anomalies in one or more body systems.[9] Extracardiac anomalies are more frequent with certain cardiac lesions, such as ventricular septal defect, tetralogy of

Table 4.6 Specific cardiac defects and the frequency of additional anomalies and aneuploidy (reproduced with permission from Gembruch and Geipel, 2005)[5]

Lesion	Aneuploidy (%)	Extracardiac anomaly (%)
Atrioventricular septal defect	35–47	30–50
Ventricular septal defect	37–48	30–37
Atrial septal defect	3	16
Tetralogy of Fallot	27	25–30
Double outlet right ventricle	12–45	19–20
Hypoplastic left heart syndrome	4	11
Truncus arteriosus communis	14–29	15–21
Transposition of great arteries	3	15–26
Coarctation of the aorta	21–29	12–20
Tricuspid atresia	2–9	15–34
Ebstein's anomaly	5–6	6
Aortic stenosis	0.2–17	13
Pulmonary stenosis/atresia	4–5	20–26

Fallot and coarctation of the aorta. There is a strong association between CHD and aneuploidy. The frequency of aneuploidy and extracardiac malformations for different types of CHD is shown in Table 4.6.

Table 4.7 Examples of structural defects associated with chromosomal abnormalities

Chromosomal defects	Associated malformations
Trisomy 21	Atrioventricular canal defect
	Duodenal atresia
Trisomy 18	Ventricular septal defect
	Exomphalos
	Micrognathia
	Congenital diaphragmatic hernia
	Rocker bottom feet
Trisomy 13	Ventricular septal defect
	Holoprosencephaly
	Facial cleft
Turner syndrome	Coarction of the aorta

Chromosomal abnormalities that are commonly reported include trisomies 21, 18 and 13 and Turner syndrome. Certain combinations of anomalies should increase suspicion regarding specific chromosomal abnormalities (Table 4.7). Certain cardiac anomalies are more frequently associated with aneuploidy, such as atrioventricular septal defect and double outlet right ventricle, and the presence of additional extracardiac anomalies further increases the risk. Karyotyping, after appropriate counselling, should be considered when a cardiac defect is detected antenatally by ultrasound. Testing for the 22q11 deletion (diGeorge syndrome) should be requested for certain cardiac anomalies; for example, tetralogy of Fallot, double outlet right ventricle and truncus arteriosus communis.

INCREASED NUCHAL TRANSLUCENCY

Increased nuchal translucency in the chromosomally normal fetus is a risk factor for CHD. One potential mechanism for the subcutaneous oedema is that narrowing of the aortic isthmus results in overperfusion of the head. The degree of risk correlates with the size of the nuchal translucency measurement. A measurement below the 95th centile is associated with a prevalence of CHD of 0.08%. In contrast, measurements of 3.5–4.4 mm and 5.5 mm or greater are associated with a prevalence of 2.89% and 19.51%, respectively.[10] In this study, 56% of cases of CHD had a nuchal translucency measurement above the 95th centile. Increased nuchal translucency was observed with all types of CHD. However, there was a stronger association with left-sided heart lesions, such as coarctation of the aorta and hypoplastic left heart syndrome (HLHS). Increased nuchal translucency therefore acts as a marker for pregnancies requiring detailed cardiac assessment.

A detailed discussion of individual cardiac defects is beyond the scope of this chapter. However, a few specific features are worth consideration. HLHS was once viewed as a universally fatal condition. Advances in surgical expertise have resulted in 5-year survival figures for surgically corrected HLHS in the region of 70%, provided that there are no complicating factors or extracardiac anomalies.[11] Ebstein's anomaly, in which the primary defect is displacement of the tricuspid valve, is associated with cardiac failure *in utero* in approximately 50% of cases. In addition, owing to increasing cardiomegaly, there is a risk of pulmonary hypoplasia. Ventricular septal defects are frequently part of more complex CHD and, if extracardiac anomalies are present, a chromosomal abnormality should be suspected. When they occur in isolation the risk of aneuploidy is much lower. Cardiac defects *per se* are not associated with fetal growth restriction. However, if there is haemodynamic compromise during fetal life, growth restriction may occur. Aortic stenosis is the lesion most commonly associated with fetal growth restriction. Approximately

6% of fetuses with CHD die *in utero*. Lesions that risk fetal death include Ebstein's anomaly, absent pulmonary valve syndrome, complete heart block, dilated or hypertrophic cardiomyopathy, cardiac tumours, pleural or pericardial effusions.

CARDIAC ANOMALIES: CONSIDERATIONS

A number of issues need to be addressed when an antenatal diagnosis of CHD is made:

- Are extracardiac anomalies present?
- Is karyotyping indicated? Should 22q11 deletion be included?
- Multidisciplinary counselling is required.
- What type of surgery is indicated?
- Will surgery result in a univentricular repair? If so, the implications for long-term cardiac function and heart transplant need to be discussed.
- Is the lesion duct-dependent: that is, will patency of the ductus arteriosus have to be maintained in the early neonatal period with intravenous prostaglandin?
- Delivery in a tertiary unit will be indicated for cases requiring immediate intervention.
- The aim should be for delivery at term unless there is fetal growth restriction or other obstetric indications.
- There is no indication for elective caesarean section on account of the cardiac defect, unless there is evidence of cardiac failure or the heart rate cannot be monitored (brady or tachy arrhythmias)
- Following a diagnosis of CHD and depending on the type of lesion, management options include termination of pregnancy, active management or palliative care.

Gastrointestinal system

The common anterior abdominal wall defects comprise gastroschisis and exomphalos. They are both amenable to antenatal diagnosis and, provided that they are isolated defects, the prognosis following early neonatal surgery is generally very good for each condition (at least 80% survival). Table 4.8 illustrates the differing features of the two conditions. The incidence of gastroschisis is approximately one in 2500–3000 live births. There is an association with teenage pregnancy, smoking and drug abuse.[12,13] The defect in the abdominal wall is to the right side of the umbilicus, through which gastrointestinal contents, usually bowel, herniate (Figure 4.8). Free loops of bowel are seen floating in the amniotic cavity on ultrasound examination. Additional structural anomalies are rare and the risk of aneuploidy is not increased.

Table 4.8   Features of gastroschisis and exomphalos

Factor	Gastroschisis	Exomphalos
Site of defect	Paraumbilical	Umbilical
Cord insertion	Left of defect	Apex of sac
Covering membrane	No	Yes
Maternal serum α-fetoprotein	Raised	May be normal
Additional abnormalities	Rare (< 10%)	30–70% (central nervous system, cardiac, renal)
Chromosomal abnormalities	Rare (< 1%)	Up to 60%
Karyotyping	Rarely indicated	Should be offered

Bowel atresia is a recognised association of gastroschisis and this can impact upon morbidity and mortality. It can be difficult to diagnose antenatally and the presence of extra-abdominal bowel dilatation on ultrasound is not predictive. Babies with gastroschisis have a tendency to be small for dates, 30% having a birth weight below the tenth centile. Serial assessment of growth, accepting the limitations of abdominal

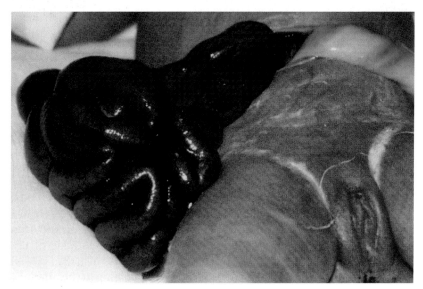

Figure 4.8 Gastroschisis: the anterior abdominal wall defect is to the right of the umbilical cord

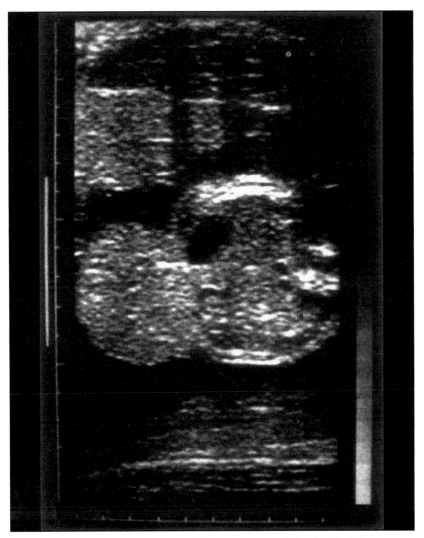

Figure 4.9 Exomphalos: ultrasound cross-section of the fetal abdomen with sac of herniated contents on the left

circumference measurements, is important. Intrauterine fetal death is a documented complication as is an increase in fetal heart rate abnormalities in labour. Serial monitoring of fetal wellbeing with umbilical and middle cerebral artery Doppler is important, before delivery at approximately 37 weeks of gestation. The aim is for a vaginal delivery unless there are other obstetric indications for caesarean section.

In contrast, exomphalos (Figure 4.9) is a midline defect in which the herniated contents are covered by a membrane and the umbilical cord inserts into the apex of the lesion. The incidence is approximately one in 5000 live births. As indicated in Table 4.8, exomphalos is associated with chromosomal and additional structural abnormalities (typically cardiac), whereas these are rare in gastroschisis. The risk of chromosomal abnormalities is highest for the small lesions that do not contain liver (67%) compared with the large defects (16%).[14] The risk of aneuploidy falls with advancing gestation, reflecting the attrition rate associated with the generally lethal anomalies that are encountered (trisomies 18 and 13). Beckwith–Wiedemann syndrome should be considered if there is associated macroglossia and macrosomia. Management involves exclusion of additional anomalies and offering karyotyping. Close fetal surveillance is required towards term as there is risk of intrauterine death (19% in one series).[15] Mode of delivery does not influence neonatal outcome and vaginal delivery is not contraindicated. In the case of a large exomphalos, caesarean section is likely to be the preferred option. Ideally, delivery should take place in a centre with access to a neonatal surgical unit.

Body stalk anomaly is a rare abdominal wall defect (one in 14 000 births) in which there is no umbilical cord and the herniated abdominal contents are attached directly to the placenta. Other anomalies are frequently present, including neural tube defects and lower limb abnormalities. It is a lethal condition and termination of pregnancy should be offered.

Congenital diaphragmatic hernia has an incidence of 0.35/1000 births in the UK. It is most commonly a posterolateral lesion located on the left side (80%). It is associated with additional structural anomalies (central nervous system, neural tube defects and exomphalos) and the risk of aneuploidy is 10–20%. Karyotyping should therefore be offered. Demonstration of fluid-filled bowel at the level of the four-chamber view of the heart on ultrasound is diagnostic, although it is a diagnosis that can easily be missed, since there can be free movement of bowel through the defect. Favourable prognostic features are a left-sided hernia and diagnosis after 24 weeks of gestation. Prognosis can, however, be difficult to predict in the antenatal period.

Duodenal atresia occurs in one in 10 000 live births. It is an isolated defect in only 50% of cases and, since up to 30% are associated with trisomy 21, karyotyping should be offered. Cardiac anomalies may be present in 10–20% of cases. The ultrasound appearance is of a 'double bubble' owing to the stomach and dilated duodenum proximal to the atresia (Figure 4.10). It should be recognised that the double bubble is not always apparent at the 20-week scan and only about 30% of cases will be suspected at this time. Polyhydramnios is often present.

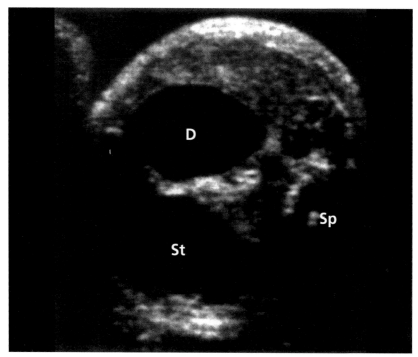

Figure 4.10 Duodenal atresia: cross-section through the fetal abdomen demonstrating 'double bubble'; D = duodenum; St = stomach; Sp = spine

Renal tract abnormalities

In the context of renal tract abnormalities, oligohydramnios indicates one of the following:

- absent kidneys
- outflow tract obstruction
- deteriorating renal function secondary to an intrinsic renal problem.

Bilateral renal agenesis is a uniformly fatal condition with an incidence of one in 3000–10 000 births. It is one of the differential diagnoses of oligohydramnios detected at a second-trimester scan (other diagnoses to consider include preterm, prelabour rupture of membranes and severe early-onset fetal growth restriction). It is a diagnosis that can be difficult to make because visualisation of the anatomy is restricted owing to oligo/anhydramnios. In addition, the adrenal glands can be mistaken for a hypoplastic kidney. Amnioinfusion can be helpful to confirm the absence of kidneys and bladder filling. Alternatively, colour flow Doppler

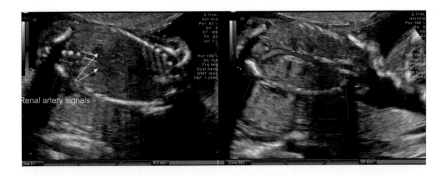

Figure 4.11 Bilateral renal arteries on colour flow (left) and power (right) Doppler

can be used to identify the presence or absence of renal arteries (Figure 4.11). It is generally a sporadic condition but it can be associated with other malformations. Fetal urine is the major source of amniotic fluid from the second trimester onwards. Amniotic fluid is essential for normal growth and development of the lungs and persistent anhydramnios from around 16 weeks onwards carries significant risk of pulmonary hypoplasia and resulting early neonatal death. Termination of pregnancy is one of the management options. In contrast, unilateral renal agenesis is usually associated with a good prognosis. The frequency of this condition is approximately one in 3000 births. It is essential to establish that the contralateral kidney is normal and that there are no additional abnormalities.

Renal tract dilatation can occur at any level from the renal pelvis to the urethra and may be unilateral or bilateral. Obstruction or reflux can result in urinary tract dilatation and differentiation of these underlying aetiologies may not be possible antenatally. A variety of grades and scales are used to describe renal pelvis dilatation (pyelectasis) and no single definition has been adopted across the board. In the fetal medicine unit at the Southern General Hospital, Glasgow, a renal pelvis measurement in the transverse plane of greater than 5 mm before 28 weeks of gestation and greater than 10 mm beyond 28 weeks of gestation requires surveillance. Pyelectasis is seen in about 2% of pregnancies and in the vast majority of cases will resolve *in utero*. Hydronephrosis can be defined as an anteroposterior diameter greater than 15 mm, with further subdivisions according to the degree of calyceal dilatation.[16]

Pelviureteric obstruction is the most common cause of hydronephrosis and is the most common lesion of the fetal urinary tract. It is more common in males and is unilateral in 80–90% of cases. Additional structural abnormalities should be excluded. The ureter is normally not

Table 4.9 Classification of cystic renal disease

Type	Potter classification	Inheritance
Infantile polycystic kidneys	Type 1	Autosomal recessive
Multicystic kidney disease	Type 2	Usually sporadic; if component of Meckel–Gruber syndrome, autosomal recessive
Adult polycystic kidney disease	Type 3	Autosomal dominant
Cystic renal dysplasia	Type 4	Sporadic

visible antenatally. Dilatation of the ureter reflects obstruction at any level within the ureter or lower urinary tract, vesicoureteral reflux or mega-ureter. If due to obstruction, the presence of a normal bladder indicates that the obstruction is at the level of the ureterovesical junction and not more distal.

Bladder dilatation is most commonly caused by obstruction at the level of the urethra, secondary to posterior urethral valves. It occurs almost exclusively in males. Back pressure leads to bilateral hydroureters and hydronephrosis. Not only do the kidneys become dysplastic as a result but growth and development of the lungs may also be compromised, owing to oligohydramnios. The condition is amenable to *in utero* therapy, vesicoamniotic shunting, which is discussed in Chapter 5. Occasionally, a bladder may become overdistended, owing to gross vesicoureteric reflux.

Cystic disease of the kidneys is classified into four types (Table 4.9). Infantile polycystic kidneys are bilaterally enlarged with a bright echogenic appearance on ultrasound. There is a spectrum of severity but, when the diagnosis is made antenatally, the prognosis is generally guarded. Adult polycystic kidney disease is, by definition, rarely diagnosed *in utero*. Multicystic kidney disease may be bilateral, unilateral or may involve only a segment of the kidney. The incidence is approximately one in 1000. The cysts are peripheral and may be multiple, varying in size. They are scattered throughout the kidney and do not communicate with each other, which can be helpful in differentiating from a hydronephrotic kidney. The size of the kidney is determined by the number and size of the cysts. If unilateral, abnormalities of the contralateral kidney are present in up to 40% of cases. Finally, renal dysplasia secondary to obstruction will lead to hyperechogenic kidneys on ultrasound. In this situation, the kidneys may be small or enlarged.

RENAL ANOMALIES: CONSIDERATIONS

- Is the liquor normal?
- If there is anhydramnios or oligohydramnios, consider renal problem, preterm, prelabour rupture of membranes, early-onset fetal growth restriction.
- Liquor volume is a surrogate marker of renal function.
- Is the renal problem unilateral or bilateral?
- If unilateral, is the other kidney normal?
- Are there additional structural anomalies; for example, central nervous system, cardiac, abdominal wall, facial?
- The incidence of karyotypic abnormality is low for truly isolated renal anomalies.
- Karyotyping should be offered in the presence of additional anomalies (risk of aneuploidy is around 12%) or if fetal therapy for lower urinary tract obstruction is being considered.
- The differential diagnosis of renal tract dilatation includes obstruction and reflux, which will be clarified by postnatal imaging.

Skeletal system

Skeletal dysplasias are a heterogeneous group of disorders which account for approximately 1% of perinatal deaths. The topic is too extensive to be covered here and the reader is directed to Chitty *et al.*[17] for a comprehensive review. Table 4.10. summarises some of the features of the

Table 4.10 Features of common skeletal dysplasias			
Type	*Mode of inheritance*	*Severity*	*Ultrasound features*
Thanatophoric dysplasia	Sporadic	Lethal	Small chest, frontal bossing, short long bones
Osteogenesis imperfecta types IIA and IIC	Autosomal dominant, most severe cases are new mutations	Lethal	Small chest, hypomineralisation, multiple rib fractures, short crumpled bones
Achondrogenesis:			
Types IA, IB	Autosomal recessive	Lethal	Hypomineralisation, very short but straight bones, small chest
Type II	Autosomal dominant/ sporadic	Lethal	
Achondroplasia	Autosomal dominant, usually a new mutation	Normal lifespan	Frontal bossing, short straight bones, polyhydramnios in third trimester

dysplasias mentioned here. Thanatophoric dysplasia is the most common skeletal dysplasia, with a frequency of one in 10 000. It usually results from a *de novo* mutation of the *FGFR3* gene and the risk of recurrence is less than 1%. It is characterised by short proximal bones and a hypoplastic 'bell-shaped' chest on ultrasound.

Osteogenesis imperfecta is a collagen disorder which results in increased bone fragility. Traditionally, four types have been described but types V–VII have recently been added to this classification. Type II presents with ultrasound features in the antenatal period. Type II is subdivided into three groups, with types IIIA and IIIC being uniformly lethal. Fractures occur *in utero*, leading to a bowed, angulated or crumpled appearance of the long bones. There may be multiple rib fractures. One characteristic ultrasound feature is indentation of the fetal skull secondary to pressure from the ultrasound transducer.

In achondrogenesis, there is severe limb shortening (the bones are straight) and hypomineralisation of the skull and vertebral bodies. The ribs are very short. Types IA, IB and II are described and all are lethal. Achondroplasia is the most common non-lethal skeletal dysplasia, with a frequency of 5–15/100 000 births. It is inherited in an autosomal dominant manner but most cases are the result of a new mutation in the *FGFR3* gene. The diagnosis can be confirmed on amniocentesis. The bones are short and straight, and may appear of normal length at the time of the 20-week scan. As a result, the diagnosis is often delayed until the third trimester, at which point there may be polyhydramnios.

SKELETAL DYSPLASIAS: CONSIDERATIONS

- Increased first-trimester nuchal translucency is a risk factor for skeletal dysplasia.
- Look at the mineralisation, length and shape of the bones.
- Bones which are short, with no other abnormality, may be constitutionally short.
- A thorough search should be made for additional anomalies, particularly cardiac, renal tract and facial anomalies.
- A small chest is suspected when the heart occupies more than one-third and the abdomen appears relatively protuberant.
- Postnatal radiological examination should be performed to ensure an accurate diagnosis and to establish recurrence risks.
- Genetic counselling is invaluable.
- Following termination of pregnancy, postmortem examination and radiological studies should be encouraged to maximise available information for future counselling.

Conclusions

Detection of a fetal structural anomaly should prompt a number of responses. A thorough structural survey must be performed to identify the presence of additional anomalies that can affect diagnosis and management and have implications for future pregnancies. Karyotyping may be indicated and appropriate counselling is essential. Discussion with a multidisciplinary team is often required to help couples make an informed decision about the subsequent management of the pregnancy. Not only is this important to help them understand the nature of the condition, it also prepares them for events that will take place in the immediate neonatal period and in the longer term. In certain circumstances, it will be appropriate to transfer care to a tertiary referral centre where there is access to neonatal surgeons. When the outlook for the pregnancy is poor and termination is the chosen option, the importance of postmortem examination should be discussed, to ensure that as much information as possible is available for counselling regarding subsequent pregnancies.

References

1. Wax JR, Bookman L, Cartin A, Pinette MG, Blackstone J. Mild fetal cerebral ventriculomegaly: diagnosis, clinical associations, and outcomes. *Obstet Gynecol Surv* 2003;58:407–14.

2. Pilu G, Falco P, Gabrielli S, Perolo S, Sandri F, Bovicelli L. The clinical significance of fetal isolated cerebral borderline ventriculomegaly: report of 31 cases and review of the literature. *Ultrasound Obstet Gynecol* 1999;14:320–6.

3. Ouahba J, Luton D, Vuillard E, Garel C, Gressens P, Blanc N, *et al.* Prenatal isolated mild ventriculomegaly: outcome in 167 cases. *BJOG* 2006;113:1072–9.

4. Laskin MD, Kingdom J, Toi Ants, Chitayat D, Ohlsson A. Perinatal and neurodevelopmental outcome with isolated fetal ventriculomegaly: a systematic review. *J Mat Fetal Neonat Med* 2005;18:289–98.

5. Hoffman JI, Christianson R. Congenital heart disease in a cohort of 19,502 births with long-term follow-up. *Am J Cardiol* 1978;42:641–7.

6. Gembruch U, Geipel A. Indication for fetal echocardiography: screening in low- and high-risk populations. In: Yagel S, Silverman NH, Gembruch U, editors. *Fetal Cardiology.* Oxford: Taylor and Francis; 2005. p. 89–106.

7. Stumpflen I, Stumpflen A, Wimmer M, Bernaschek G. Effect of detailed fetal echocardiography as part of routine prenatal ultrasonographic screening on detection of congenital heart disease. *Lancet* 1996;348:854–7.

8. Carvalho JS. Early prenatal diagnosis of major congenital heart defects. *Curr Opin Obstet Gynecol* 2001;13:155–9.

9. Wallgren EI, Landtman B, Rapola J. Extracardiac malformations associated with congenital heart disease. *Eur J Cardiol* 1978;7:15–24.

10. Hyett J, Perdu M, Sharland G, Snijders R, Nicolaides KH. Using fetal nuchal translucency to screen for major congenital cardiac defects at 10-14 weeks gestation: population based cohort study. *BMJ* 1999;318:81–5.

11. O'Kelly SW, Bove EL. Hypoplastic left heart syndrome. Terminal care is not the only option. *BMJ* 1997;314:87–8.

12. Tan KH, Kilby MD, Whittle MJ, Beattie BR, Booth IW, Botting BJ. Congenital anterior abdominal wall defects in England and Wales, 1987–1993: retrospective analysis of OPCS data. *Br Med J* 1996;313:903–6.

13. Morrison JJ, Chitty LS, Peebles D, Rodeck CH. Recreational drugs and fetal gastroschisis: maternal hair analysis in the periconceptional period during pregnancy. *BJOG* 2005;112:1022–5.

14. Nyberg DA, Fitzsimmons J, Mack LH, Hughes M, Pretorius DH, Hickok D, *et al.* Chromosomal abnormalities in fetuses with omphalocoele: significance of omphalocoele contents. *J Ultrasound Med* 1989;8:299–308.

15. Fratelli N, Papageorghiou AT, Bhide A, Sharma A, Okoye B, Thilaganathan B. Outcome of antenatally diagnosed abdominal wall defects. *Ultrasound Obstet Gynecol* 2007;30:266–70.

16. Grignon A, Filion R, Filiatrault D, Robitaille P, Homsy Y, Boutin H, *et al.* Urinary tract dilatation in utero: classification and clinical applications. *Radiology* 1986;160:645–7.

17. Chitty LS, Wilson L, Griffin D. Fetal skeletal abnormalities. In: Rodeck CK, Whittle MJ, editors. *Fetal Medicine Basic Science and Clinical Practice*. Edinburgh: Churchill Livingstone; 2009. p. 478–513.

5 Fetal therapy

Historical aspects

Treatment of the fetus *in utero* has been a possibility for obstetricians since the 1960s. This was a time when the dawn of a new branch of medicine, perinatal medicine, became a reality through the contributions of obstetricians such as Professor Ian Donald in Glasgow and Dr AW Liley in New Zealand. Their research on the development of ultrasound and amniocentesis in rhesus sensitisation enabled doctors to treat the fetus as a patient. Since then, other milestones in the creation of this branch of medicine have been Professor GC Liggins' work in the 1970s on the maternal administration of corticosteroids to prevent respiratory distress syndrome and the practical and laboratory genetic techniques for prenatal diagnosis in the first trimester of pregnancy throughout the 1980s.

The key to the success of attempts at fetal diagnosis and therapy has been the continued improvement in fetal imaging techniques, mainly with high-resolution ultrasound techniques and the use of ultrafast magnetic resonance imaging. In the future, rapid progress is likely to be made in real time three-dimensional ultrasound procedures and, together with advances in minimal-access surgical techniques, the concept of providing true fetal treatment is a real possibility in the years ahead.

The main clinical areas of focus as regards potential fetal therapy have been prematurity, fetal growth restriction, fetal malformations and specific genetic conditions. The main types of fetal therapy that were introduced include preventive therapy, transplacental treatment, perinatal management of the fetus with a malformation and invasive fetal procedures.

Preventive therapy

Preventive therapy involves public health education, giving general advice on maternal health and diet, with a specific focus on smoking cessation and limitation of alcohol intake during pregnancy.[1] Certain fetal malformations, such as neural tube defects, warrant specific consideration. The birth prevalence of neural tube defects varies geographically, with greater incidence in some parts of the UK.[2,3] Women who have had one infant with a neural tube defect have a risk of recurrence some ten-fold greater than women in general, about 3–4%. It has been clearly shown that the majority of defects can be prevented by increasing maternal folic acid intake over the time of conception and through the first 12 weeks of pregnancy.[4] The recommended supplementary dose of folic acid is 400 micrograms in addition to the average dietary intake of 0.2 mg daily. Health authorities, hospital and primary care trusts are trying to increase public awareness of this important preventive strategy through promotional materials in general practitioner surgeries, hospital clinics and in pharmacists' shops.[1] A higher dose of 5 mg daily is recommended for women with insulin-dependent diabetes, epilepsy and women who have had a previous pregnancy affected with a neural tube defect.

Other prepregnancy advice, such as avoidance of drugs and potential teratogens, should be widely given, as should specific measures such as rubella vaccination to those at risk and strict control of the blood sugar in women with insulin-dependent diabetes.

Fetal therapy in women who have inborn errors of metabolism can be considered in a number of ways. The maternal metabolic disorder may be the primary disease and an adverse fetal effect secondary. Optimal maternal care is then required for the wellbeing of both the mother and her fetus. This is the case in maternal phenylketonuria and Wilson's disease, where the fetus is the passive victim of the maternal metabolic derangement. In these conditions, the primary goal of maternal therapy is to optimise the fetal environment to minimise the risk of fetal damage in an otherwise unaffected fetus.

Indirect (transplacental) fetal therapy

MEDICAL TREATMENT AND FETAL PHARMACOKINETICS

The mechanism for medical fetal therapy involves the transplacental passage of substances via the maternal circulation. This chiefly involves administration of a drug, hormone or vitamin to the mother. Drugs mainly move across the placenta by simple diffusion but the process is dependent on the chemical properties and concentration gradients of the free drug. Drug transfer is greater in late gestation but pathological conditions causing inflammation, hypoxia, vascular degeneration or separation of the placenta can affect uteroplacental blood flow and thus transfer of the drug. Like the liver, the placenta is capable of drug biotransformation and some drugs may only cross the placenta after this has occurred. For most drugs that cross the placenta, fetal levels reach 50–100% of maternal serum concentrations. However, once the levels reach steady state, fetal serum levels can be higher than maternal levels. The total time exposed to a drug and its metabolites is more important than the rate of transplacental transport. As fetal systems are not fully developed, the excretion of drugs is much slower than in the adult. The main routes of elimination involve the placenta and fetal urine. In early pregnancy, the primary route of elimination is by placental transfer to the maternal circulation, whereas in later gestation drugs are eliminated into the amniotic fluid via the fetal kidneys.

CONGENITAL ADRENAL HYPERPLASIA

Congenital adrenal hyperplasia (CAH) was the first example of an inborn error of metabolism inherited by the fetus that can be treated *in utero* with prevention of the malformation as the primary goal. This disorder has been linked to chromosome 6. The clinical spectrum of disease associated with CAH ranges from the life-threatening wasting variety to mild virilisation in males or ambiguous genitalia in females. Prominent clitoromegaly with labial fusion can lead to incorrect gender assignment at birth.

Since CAH is an autosomal recessive condition and only the females will be affected by the anomaly, the birth defect risk is one in eight. Virilisation of the female fetus may occur during weeks 10–16 of gestation and therefore preventive *in utero* therapy needs to be started before determination of gender or disease status. This can be achieved by suppressing the fetal adrenal gland by maternal administration of dexamethasone. It has been recommended that maternal dexamethasone therapy be initiated as early as 5 weeks of gestation using a dose of 20 micrograms/kg/day.[5] *In utero* treatment can now be targeted to a female fetus using noninvasive prenatal diagnosis by employing the laboratory techniques which can determine fetal sexing from free fetal DNA in a maternal serum sample.[6] If the fetus is an affected female, maternal therapy should be continued until delivery. Despite these measures, one-third of these neonates still exhibit some degree of virilisation.

FETAL DYSRHYTHMIAS

The majority of disturbances of fetal cardiac rhythm are noted either incidentally during auscultation of the fetal heart or during an ultrasound examination. The type of arrhythmia can be established using fetal M-mode echocardiography and duplex-pulsed and colour Doppler (Figure 5.1). The most common fetal dysrhythmia is supraventricular tachycardia (SVT) followed by atrial flutter. SVT is most often caused by reciprocating or atrioventricular re-entrant tachycardia. The ventricular rate is always rapid (240–260 beats/minute) and can lead to fetal hydrops. The need for fetal therapy is based upon a number of factors including gestational age, presence or absence of hydrops and the estimated duration of the tachycardia. Immature fetuses with hydrops are thus the most obvious

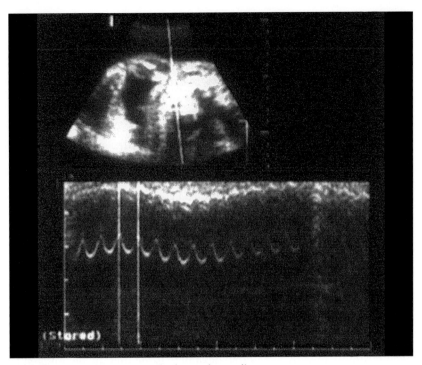

Figure 5.1 Fetal supraventricular tachycardia

candidates for anti-arrhythmic treatment. The primary aim is to convert the rhythm back to normal *in utero* and to deliver the fetus in normal sinus rhythm at or near term.[7]

In SVT, digoxin is usually favoured for the non-hydropic fetus and flecainide for the hydropic fetus because of its better passage across the placenta. Maternal oral digoxin therapy is successful in approximately 60% of cases. The dose required is 0.5–1.0 mg daily. Flecainide is given at a dose of 100 mg twice daily. Fetuses that do not respond to either of these drugs may be candidates for direct fetal therapy in an attempt to achieve medical cardioversion of SVT using adenosine directly injected into the fetal umbilical or hepatic vein.[8] This is usually a last resort in severely hydropic fetuses with tachycardia resistant to transplacental therapy.

Non-hydropic cases can be treated as outpatients, whereas hydropic cases require inpatient treatment. Evaluation and treatment should be performed in a tertiary fetal medicine centre. However, unless obstetric complications occur and the rhythm disturbance fails to respond to treatment, local delivery can be considered.[9]

The types of rhythm disturbance causing fetal bradycardia include sinus bradycardia, blocked atrial ectopic beats and complete heart block.

Examination using M-mode and Doppler echocardiography aids the differentiation. Atrial ectopic beats usually resolve spontaneously and reassuring counselling is recommended. Fetuses with complete heart block should have a detailed cardiac ultrasound examination to look for evidence of associated CHD and the mother should be checked for the presence of maternal autoantibodies, namely anti-SSA/Ro and anti-SSB/La. The detection of such antibodies is important, since there is potential fetal therapy in the form of maternal dexamethasone 4 mg daily. This has had limited success and an attempt to run a European multicentre trial was abandoned owing to poor enrolment.[10] When fetal hydrops is present, the prognosis is poor and has not been improved by fetal therapy with agents such as salbutamol and direct fetal pacing. Fetuses with complete heart block should be delivered in a tertiary fetal medicine centre with easy access to a paediatric cardiology service. The method of delivery is normally elective caesarean section in view of the inability to monitor the fetal heart rate in labour.

Invasive fetal therapy

ULTRASOUND-GUIDED THERAPY

The continuing improvements in ultrasound technology have permitted the fetal medicine specialist to examine the fetus in a similar way that other medical practitioners examine extrauterine patients. A variety of investigations can be undertaken and, in certain conditions, direct fetal treatment can be instigated in an attempt to improve the neonatal prognosis. All these developments involve multidisciplinary teamwork, which begins with detailed counselling before any planned intervention. In view of the complexities of such cases, invasive fetal therapy is usually performed in specialised tertiary referral centres where couples can be counselled and receive treatment from the members of the multidisciplinary perinatal team.

Prior to embarking on fetal therapy, a detailed assessment of both the maternal and fetal condition is required. The views and wishes of the prospective parents must be entirely respected. Factors such as the need to exclude chromosomal abnormalities will be discussed before embarking on fetal therapy. The advantages and disadvantages of proposed therapies need to be discussed in great detail and in certain circumstances other members of the perinatal team will be involved. This will permit the parents to be fully aware of the potential neonatal prognosis and whether alternative strategies may offer other management options. It is crucial that such discussions take place in an unhurried, calm environment and that the parents are given ample time to ask questions and meet with other members of the perinatal team.

INTRAVASCULAR TRANSFUSION FOR RHESUS DISEASE

Intrauterine transfusion was the original fetal therapy described by Liley in the 1960s. He described intraperitoneal transfusion via a catheter placed under fluoroscopic control into the fetal peritoneal cavity (Figure 5.2). Since then, there have been continued advances in this area of fetal therapy and the contribution of these procedures to the reduction of perinatal mortality due to rhesus disease is illustrated in Figure 5.3.

Assessment of at-risk pregnancies

HISTORY AND ANTIBODIES

A number of factors are taken into consideration when deciding upon the likely need for and timing of fetal blood transfusion. Maternal past obstetric history and neonatal history of top-up or exchange transfusion are both important since, if a subsequent pregnancy is affected, this is likely to occur at an earlier gestation. Maternal antibody quantification gives an indication of the progression of disease, with the trend in rise of antibody levels being as important as a fixed cut-off level. Paternal zygosity is also important. If the father is heterozygous, it is important to establish the fetal blood group. This can now be achieved by sending a sample of maternal serum where noninvasive prenatal diagnosis of the fetal blood type using the free fetal DNA techniques can be performed in one of the national reference laboratories.[11] It is generally accepted that the critical titre for anti-D in a first affected pregnancy is 1/32.[12] An anti-D

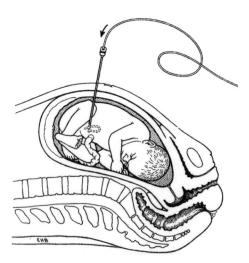

Figure 5.2 Intraperitoneal transfusion

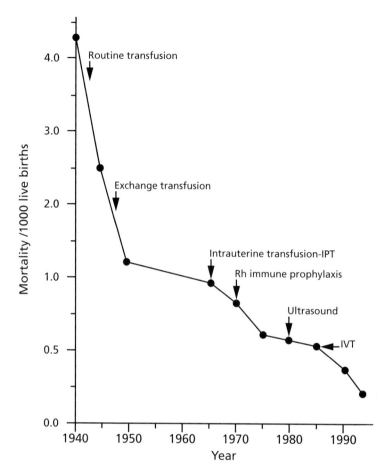

Figure 5.3 Developments in the management of rhesus disease
IPT = intraperitoneal transfusion
IVT = intravascular transfusion; Rh = rhesus

quantification less than 4 iu/ml is unlikely to be associated with haemolytic disease of the newborn but there is a moderate risk between 4 iu/ml and 15 iu/ml. However, it is not only the cut-off point that is important but the trend of rise in antibody quantification.

ULTRASOUND

Ultrasound surveillance to detect early signs of fetal hydrops (Figure 5.4a,b) is important. Amniocentesis has traditionally been the next line of investigation following a rise in maternal antibodies. This technique allows measurement of the bilirubin concentration (delta OD450) in amniotic fluid and gives an indirect estimate of fetal haemolysis. The level is plotted on the Liley curve (Figure 5.5) and this gives an estimation of risk depending upon which Liley zone the level corresponds to. Values for OD450 in the lower zone indicated a fetus with mild or no haemolytic disease while those in the upper zone indicated severe haemolytic disease with fetal death probable in 7–10 days. The Liley curve became the cornerstone of management for the

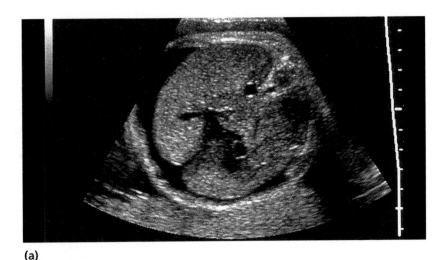

(a)

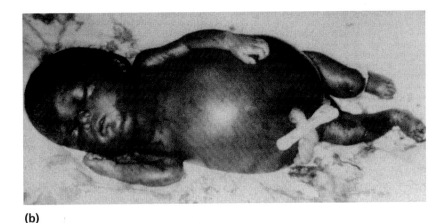

(b)

Figure 5.4 Hydrops fetalis (a) transverse section of fetal abdomen showing fetal ascites; (b) after birth

OD

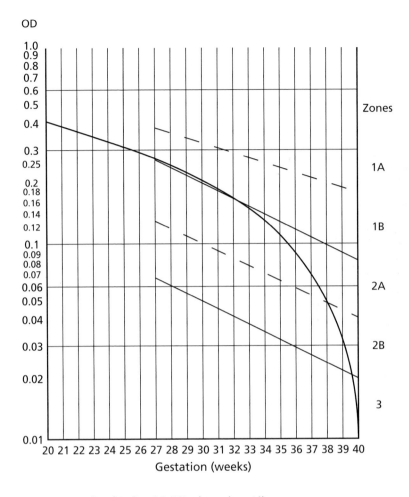

Figure 5.5 Levels of Delta OD450 plotted on Liley curve

pregnant woman with red-cell alloimmunisation. However, in recent years there has been a loss of faith in amniocentesis as a useful tool for predicting fetal disease, especially at early gestations. Amniocentesis also carries the risk of aggravating maternal sensitisation and therefore the role of noninvasive tests has been explored.

Middle cerebral artery peak systolic velocity measurement is one such technique. The underlying theory is that the anaemic fetus has a reduced blood viscosity and increased cardiac output, both of which lead to measurable increase in peak systolic velocity (PSV) assessed by Doppler ultrasound (Figure 5.6a,b). Current evidence indicates that a PSV of greater than 1.5 MoM has 100% sensitivity in the prediction of moderate

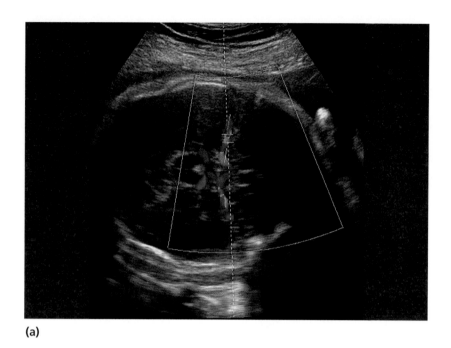

(a)

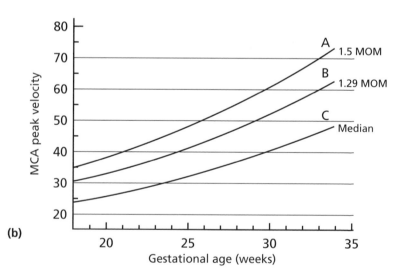

(b)

Figure 5.6 Measurement of middle cerebral artery peak systolic velocity:
(a) Doppler ultrasound; (b) displayed graphically;
A = moderate to severe anaemia; B = mild anaemia;
C = no anaemia; MCA = middle cerebral artery;
MOM = multiples of the median

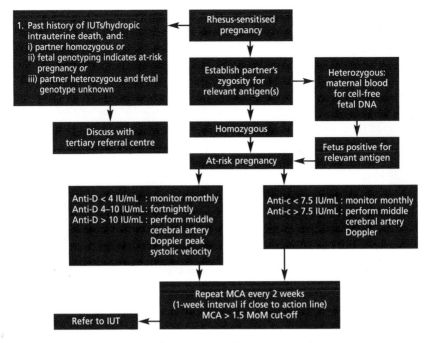

Figure 5.7 Management of rhesus-sensitised pregnancies; IU international units; IUT intrauterine transfusion; MCA middle cerebral artery; MoM multiples of the median

to severe anaemia and has now gained acceptance in clinical practice.[13] The technique has been subjected to a randomised clinical trial which demonstrated clear advantages in favour of the noninvasive procedure.[14] If intrauterine transfusion is deemed necessary, this should be performed in a tertiary referral centre with fetal medicine specialists experienced in the technique. The mother must be counselled about the nature of the procedure, the requirement for repeated transfusions and the potential complications. An algorithm for the management of rhesus-sensitised pregnancies is shown in Figure 5.7.[15]

FETAL INTRAUTERINE TRANSFUSION

Intrauterine transfusion is an aseptic technique carried out under ultrasound guidance. The mother is fasted, sedated and given antibiotics to cover the procedure. Steroids are given to promote pulmonary maturity once fetal viability is reached. The intravascular route has superseded the intraperitoneal route, which was the technique used for the first intrauterine transfusions. While the technique is simpler than an intravascular transfusion, the red cells have to be absorbed from the peritoneal cavity

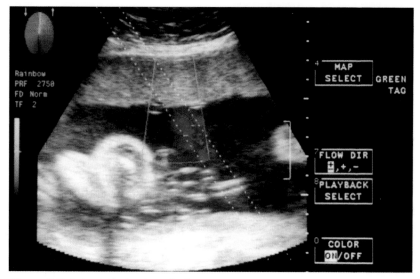

Figure 5.8 Intravascular transfusion

into the fetal circulation and, hence, the response to treatment is delayed. In current clinical practice, intraperitoneal transfusion is confined to those cases requiring transfusion at very early gestations. Some of the technical aspects of intrauterine transfusion are shown in Figure 5.7.[15]

A pre-procedure scan with colour-flow mapping is carried out to establish the site for transfusion. A 20-gauge spinal needle and needle guide are used to gain access to the desired vessel (Figure 5.8). In general, the umbilical vein at the placental cord insertion is chosen and free loops of cord are avoided, to minimise the risk of the needle being dislodged by fetal activity. The cord root is most accessible if the placenta is anterior. Posterior placental locations can be more difficult to reach. It may be necessary to give the transfusion via the intrahepatic portion of the umbilical vein but this is dependent on fetal position. Occasionally, it is necessary to paralyse the fetus with vecuronium 0.25 mg/kg.

With the needle in the vessel, a 1–2 ml sample is taken to check the fetal blood parameters, including haematocrit direct Coombs test and karyotype. A dedicated laboratory team is required for the transfusion procedure; 2 ml of (0.9%) physiological saline is flushed through the needle to establish flow in the vessel and the transfusion is commenced while the fetal haematocrit is being measured. O-negative, irradiated, cytomegalovirus-negative packed red cells are transfused. A donor haematocrit in the region of 70% is preferable, as this reduces the volume of transfusion. The laboratory staff calculate the volume of blood to be transfused using a formula incorporating the fetal haematocrit, the

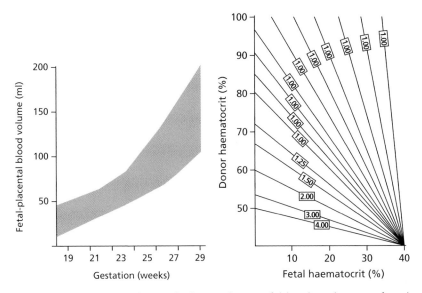

Figure 5.9 Graphs used to calculate volume of blood to be transfused: (left) fetal placental blood volume; (right) fetal haematocrit

haematocrit of the donor blood and the fetoplacental volume (Figure 5.9). Once the required amount has been transfused, the vessel is flushed with 2 ml 0.9% physiological saline and a post-transfusion haematocrit is checked. If this is in the region of 40–45%, the transfusion is discontinued. The injection of blood into the vessel results in turbulence that can be demonstrated ultrasonically. The fetal heart rate is checked intermittently during the procedure. The mother returns to the ward and cardiotocography is carried out. An ultrasound scan is performed the following day and if a satisfactory haematocrit has been reached transfusions are repeated at fortnightly intervals until 34 weeks of gestation (Figure 5.10). Induction of labour or caesarean section is organised soon thereafter.

Emergency delivery by caesarean section is sometimes required if the fetus sustains a prolonged bradycardia, so the labour ward staff and the neonatal team should always be informed when transfusions are taking place. The perinatal mortality rate is 1.6–2.0%.[16]

FETAL AND NEONATAL ALLOIMMUNE THROMBOCYTOPENIA

Fetal and neonatal alloimmune thrombocytopenia (FNAIT) is the platelet equivalent of rhesus disease. It is caused by maternal immunoglobulin G

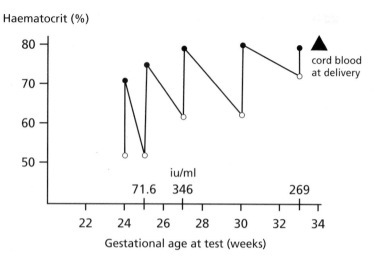

Figure 5.10 Timing of transfusions until delivery

alloantibodies, which cross the placenta and are directed against human platelet antigens (HPA) on fetal platelets. In white races, the immunodominant antigen is HPA-1a, which is responsible for approximately 85% of cases of FNAIT. FNAIT is uncommon, occurring at a rate of one in 1000–2000 live births. Infant morbidity and mortality, however, are high, with intracranial haemorrhage being the most severe complication. This occurs in 10–30% of neonates affected by fetal alloimmune thrombocytopenia and is thought to have occurred *in utero* in 50% of these cases.[17] Therapy aimed at preventing this complication must therefore be instituted antenatally.

Maternal therapy, in the form of weekly intravenous immunoglobulin at a dose of 1g/kg, has been reported as being successful.[18] The direct therapeutic approach requires fetal blood sampling and serial platelet transfusions if the fetal platelet count is less than 50 000. This needs to be repeated every 7–10 days but is a more hazardous procedure than transfusion for rhesus disease, owing to the risk of exsanguination from the site of blood sampling. Over the last 15 years, there has been a gradual change in antenatal treatment, from an invasive management protocol to a less invasive and noninvasive approach. However, controversy still exists regarding the optimal management strategy.[19]

Fetal shunting procedures

FETAL URINARY TRACT OBSTRUCTION

Fetal obstructive uropathies may involve the upper and lower urinary

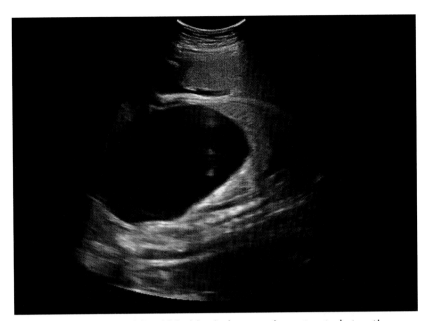

Figure 5.11 Distended fetal bladder in lower urinary tract obstruction

tract. *In utero* treatment is only considered if there is a bladder obstruction, usually as a result of posterior urethral valves in a male fetus. The incidence of obstructive uropathy is approximately 1/2000 pregnancies. This condition is now more commonly referred to as lower urinary tract

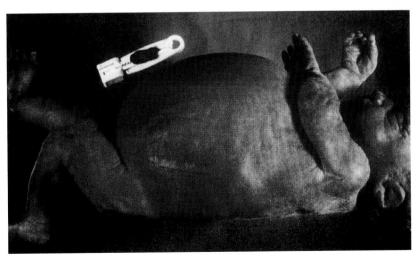

Figure 5.12 A fetus with 'prune belly' syndrome

obstruction (LUTO). Typically, this produces an enlarged fetal bladder, bilateral hydronephrosis and decreased amniotic fluid volume (Figure 5.11). In its most severe form, a condition known as 'prune belly' syndrome arises (Figure 5.12) with high mortality from pulmonary hypoplasia.

Antenatal assessment

When a diagnosis of LUTO is made, further investigations should be considered. It is important that an experienced sonographer determines the fetal sex, assesses liquor volume and renal architecture and looks for other anomalies. Fetal karyotyping should also be offered. Assessment of fetal renal function has been attempted, mainly through measurement of electrolytes in the fetal urine by performing vesicoentesis. The importance of serial sampling is well described and must be performed at set intervals for the information to retain its predictive value. It is recommended that the bladder be drained over 48–72 hours and measurements of sodium, chloride, osmolality, calcium, 2-microglobulin and total protein carried out. The urine thresholds for selecting fetuses for intrauterine therapy are shown in Table 5.1. A minimum of three bladder drainages provides optimal predictive value. However, a systematic review of the clinical usefulness of fetal urinary analysis in predicting neonatal renal function concluded that there was insufficient evidence to continue the practice of providing fetal therapy on the basis of electrolyte results.[20]

Fetal therapy for LUTO

Fetal therapy for LUTO involves the insertion of a catheter or shunt into the fetal bladder to drain urine into the amniotic cavity, thus bypassing the obstruction and preventing fetal kidney damage. The early use of double 'pigtail' catheters placed into the fetal bladder met with highly variable success rates. The criteria for intervention were highly variable and evaluation of the fetus before treatment was minimal in most cases.

Table 5.1	Urine thresholds for selecting fetuses for intrauterine therapy
Sample	*Threshold*
Sodium	< 100 mg/dl
Chloride	< 90 mg/dl
Osmolality	< 200 mOsm/l
Calcium	< 8 mg/dl
β-2-microglobulin	< 6 mg/dl
Total protein	< 20 mg/dl

The success of intervention for LUTO remains controversial. A review of the five largest series reported survival after intervention in 47% and shunt-related complications occurred in 45% of cases. Although not all fetuses had oligohydramnios, of those that did, 56% died despite shunting. Failure to restore amniotic fluid was associated with 100% mortality. Vesicoamniotic shunting in cases of poor urinary function prognosis was associated with postnatal renal insufficiency in 87.5% of cases and, whereas intervention did improve the chances of survival, it did not alter the renal outcomes. These findings have been illustrated in a follow-up study, which suggested that a significant number of fetuses with so-called good prognostic signs still had a high rate of underlying primary renal dysplasia.[21] In view of the paucity of data supporting bladder shunting for LUTO[22] to improve neonatal renal function, a randomised clinical trial (PLUTO)[23] has been commenced. This trial is a randomised, controlled trial designed to investigate the role of vesico-amniotic shunting in babies with moderate or severe LUTO.

VESICOAMNIOTIC SHUNTING PROCEDURE

The best results are obtained using the Rodeck-style double pigtailed shunt. The optimal site for shunt placement is midway between the pubic ramus and the insertion of the umbilical cord. The most common complication is shunt displacement, which often leads to urinary ascites. This can be treated by the insertion of a further shunt to drain the urinary ascites. Shunt placement is performed under simultaneous ultrasound control with the chosen site on the maternal abdomen infiltrated with local anaesthesia. Maternal antibiotic therapy is also administered before and after the procedure.

There is agreement among fetal medicine centres performing these invasive procedures that collaborative data should be collected so that the natural history of such conditions and their long-term morbidity and mortality can be accurately defined. This is also an aim of the PLUTO study[23] where nonrandomised patients will be entered into a registry which will ultimately inform both patients and clinicians regarding the natural history of LUTO. A recent review of congenital urinary tract obstruction provides further reading in this area.[24]

FETAL PLEURAL EFFUSIONS

Fetal pleural effusions occur in approximately one in 10 000 pregnancies and may be either primary (hydrothorax), usually as a result of chylothorax, or secondary as a result of aneuploidy or infection (Figure 5.13). They may also lead to nonimmune hydrops. The first step in detecting a pleural effusion should be to determine whether it is primary

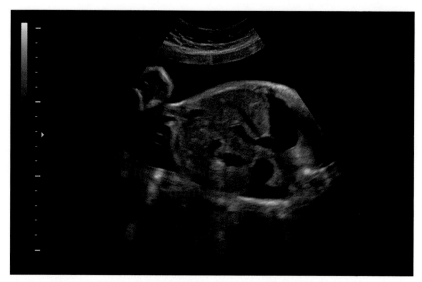

Figure 5.13 Bilateral pleural effusions in a fetus with chylothorax

or secondary. Primary fetal hydrothorax is a diagnosis of exclusion and investigations are similar to those for nonimmune hydrops: maternal serology to exclude congenital infections (toxoplasmosis, rubella, cytomegalovirus, syphilis, herpes and parvovirus B19); blood type and antibody screen to rule out immune hydrops; Kleihauer test to exclude fetomaternal haemorrhage and Doppler evaluation of the middle cerebral artery peak systolic velocity to exclude fetal anaemia. As with other potential fetal therapeutic procedures, a detailed search for other anomalies must be made using high-resolution ultrasound and including fetal echocardiography. The couple should have the findings explained and fetal karyotyping should be offered. At the time of karyotyping, an aspiration of the pleural fluid can also be performed and this may shed some light on the underlying aetiology. The presence of high mono-nuclear counts is diagnostic of a chylothorax.

Primary fetal hydrothorax can regress, remain stable or worsen. Critical factors determining the eventual neonatal outcome are the aetiology, presence of hydrops, the gestational age at presentation and the ability to offer fetal therapy. The overall perinatal mortality is approximately 50% and associated anomalies are found in 40% of cases. Spontaneous regression is estimated to occur in 20% of cases.

If the effusions are seen before 32 weeks, conservative management is most appropriate if there is no evidence of hydrops and if the effusion is not increasing in severity. In approximately 50% of cases, fetal hydrops is present at the initial presentation or is seen to develop during the time of

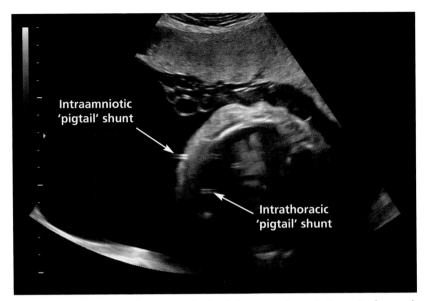

Intraamniotic 'pigtail' shunt

Intrathoracic 'pigtail' shunt

Figure 5.14 Pleuroamniotic shunt in fetal thorax and amniotic cavity (arrows)

observation. When hydrops is noted, fetal therapy should be discussed. This consists of thoracentesis and/or placement of a thoracoamniotic shunt (Figures 5.14 and 5.15). The type of shunt used depends on the gestational age of the fetus, the larger Rodeck-style shunts being suitable for the larger

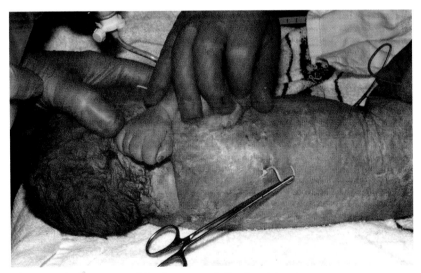

Figure 5.15 Neonate with pleuroamniotic shunt in place

fetus, whereas the Somatex® shunts are more suitable for the fetus of a lower gestational age. Placement of the shunt is performed under direct ultrasound guidance, using the same technique as is used in bladder shunts. In cases of bilateral effusions, shunts are required on both sides. The outcome after shunting is dramatically influenced by the presence of nonimmune hydrops, with perinatal survival of 70–100% in its absence compared with 45–65% survival in fetuses with the condition.[25] A systematic review of pleuroamniotic shunting has also been conducted.[26]

Such fetal therapy may reverse fetal hydrops and polyhydramnios, thus reducing the risk of preterm delivery. The extent to which it improves lung development and prevents pulmonary hypoplasia is unknown. Again, few long-term follow-up data are available in terms of neonatal and childhood survival and morbidity; prospective evaluation is required. A new form of fetal therapy for hydrothorax is the creation of pleurodesis by the injection of the sclerosant OK-432 into the pleural space.[27] Further research in the use of this technique is awaited.

Procedures used to alter the amount of amniotic fluid

AMNIOINFUSION

Amnioinfusion has been used both as a diagnostic and therapeutic procedure. Often, it is difficult to be clear whether the mother has undergone preterm prelabour rupture of the membranes (PPROM) or if the oligohydramnios has a primary fetal or placental aetiology. Despite these pathophysiological uncertainties, pregnancies complicated by oligohydramnios at an early gestational age have a poor prognosis, owing to the strong chance of pulmonary hypoplasia developing. If there is a calculated high probability of associated pulmonary hypoplasia, termination of pregnancy should be discussed. However, it is well known that ultrasound predictors of pulmonary hypoplasia are extremely poor and this is further complicated by the fact that obtaining good views of the fetal anatomy and establishing the aetiology is made even more difficult because of the absence of amniotic fluid, which provides the normal acoustic window.

Transabdominal instillation of artificial amniotic fluid is a useful technique used to improve the ultrasound image.[28] Ringer's solution is usually used, with approximately 100–200 ml being infused, depending on the gestational age. The procedure is undertaken under simultaneous ultrasound guidance using a 20-gauge needle and a three-way tap. Continuous turbulence of the instilled fluid should be visualised.

The procedure may unmask pre-existing PPROM and this can influence the counselling given to the prospective parents. It is unclear whether repeated amnioinfusion can prevent pulmonary hypoplasia and the potential maternal complications of acute infection must not be underestimated.

AMNIODRAINAGE

Amniodrainage is performed when there is clinical polyhydramnios, which is associated with considerable excess perinatal mortality because of the association between fetal structural anomaly, uteroplacental perfusion abnormality and preterm labour. Medical therapies to reduce liquor volume have included the use of prostaglandin synthetase inhibitors, such as indomethacin. The potential adverse effects are both maternal, in terms of gastrointestinal irritation, fluid retention and coagulopathies, and fetal, in terms of premature closure of the ductus arteriosus and cerebral vasoconstriction. The effects are dose-dependent and different dosage regimens are used in the USA (200–400 mg/day) compared with 75–150 mg daily in the UK. The length of time from administration of the drug to it having an effect on amniotic fluid volume is a further disadvantage of medical amnioreduction, since there may be no noticeable clinical effect for 7–10 days.

Amnioreduction by repeated intermittent amniocentesis can be of benefit in the management of polyhydramnios by reducing intra-amniotic pressure. Repeated amniocenteses do, however, carry an increased risk of infection, preterm delivery and placental abruption.

Amniodrainage has been one of the key therapies used in the management of twin–twin transfusion syndrome (TTTS). This complication is described in greater detail in Chapter 9. More recently, fetoscopic laser coagulation of chorionic plate vessels has been introduced. The results of laser therapy are discussed later in this chapter. The publication of the only randomised clinical trial in TTTS has showed clear benefit in terms of number of survivors and percentage of neonatal neurodevelopmental morbidity and hence selective laser ablation of anastomosing vessels is now the preferred fetal therapy for TTTS.

'Open' fetal surgery

Although most fetal malformations diagnosed antenatally are best managed in the neonatal period, a few severe abnormalities may be better treated by correction before birth. Extensive research using animal models of fetal conditions, together with technological advances, has led to a growth in human fetal surgery, although at present only a few life-threatening malformations have been successfully corrected. The main obstacles are rupture of the fetal membranes and control of preterm labour.

The types of fetal malformations that have the potential to be treated by fetal surgery are listed in Box 5.1.

CONGENITAL DIAPHRAGMATIC HERNIA

The main experience in human fetal cases has been with congenital diaphragmatic hernia (CDH). This condition occurs in 1/2000 to 1/5000 live births. The overall prognosis is dependent upon when and to what extent viscera are herniated into the fetal chest leading to pulmonary hypoplasia (Figure 5.16) as the degree of pulmonary hypoplasia is the

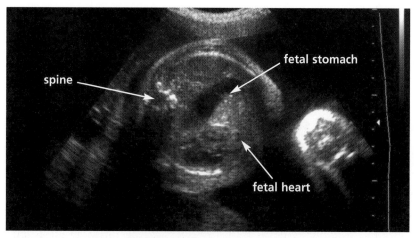

Figure 5.16 Congenital diaphragmatic hernia (CDH): transverse section through the fetal thorax demonstrating a left-sided CDH with the fetal stomach displacing the fetal heart to the right

most significant determinant of mortality in CDH. Currently, up to 30% of babies with isolated CDH die from the consequences of lung hypoplasia and/or pulmonary hypertension.[29] The initial pioneering work in this area was performed by Michael Harrison and his team in San Francisco. The challenge for clinicians being able to offer fetal therapy in CDH remains in the field of prediction of neonatal outcome. The ultimate prognosis depends on fetal lung size, which can be measured by the so-called lung-to-head ratio. Much research in the application of predictive techniques has been reported.[30] This has led to workers on both sides of the Atlantic developing techniques to achieve tracheal occlusion, with the aim of stimulating fetal lung growth *in utero*. Tracheal occlusion has gone through the stages of laparotomy, hysterotomy, neck dissection and tracheal clipping, uterine exposure and endoscopic tracheal dissection and clipping through multiple cannulae.[31] In Europe, the Fetal Endoscopic Tracheal Occlusion (FETO) Task Force has developed special instruments for a clinical technique via 3.3-mm percutaneous access. The FETO technique ultimately places a detachable balloon at the carina in the fetal trachea. Currently, the procedure is being performed in four European centres. It is carried out under locoregional anaesthesia with fetal paralysis, with reversal of the occlusion either by ultrasound-guided puncture or by fetoscopy. FETO would appear to be a useful form of fetal therapy for CDH with encouraging initial results.[32] Funding has now become available for a randomised trial, the results of which will be eagerly awaited.

FETAL LUNG LESIONS

Two common fetal lung lesions amenable to fetal therapy are congenital cystadenomatoid malformation (CCAM) and bronchopulmonary sequestration. Bronchopulmonary sequestration can usually be distinguished from CCAM by the detection of systemic arterial blood supply arising from the aorta on colour-flow Doppler. The largest reported series are from Philadelphia.[33] With an experience of over 500 cases, they have found that the overall prognosis depends on the size of the thoracic mass and the secondary physiological derangement. Larger masses lead to mediastinal shift, pulmonary hypoplasia, polyhydramnios and fetal hydrops and, ultimately, fetal death. Smaller lesions can cause neonatal respiratory distress and the smallest masses may be asymptomatic until later in childhood.

The complexity of counselling couples regarding the prognosis for these conditions is confounded by the not infrequent finding that some of the large fetal tumours seen in fetal life regress in size on serial ultrasound examinations and many non-cystic bronchopulmonary sequestrations dramatically decrease in size before birth and may not need treatment after birth. In view of the wide spectrum of outcomes for fetuses and neonates with lung lesions, it is critical that these cases are referred to a regional fetal medicine centre, where accurate prognostic information can be gathered to provide counselling. If the situation is severe, with the presence of other associated life-threatening malformations, or if the mother is sick with 'mirror' or 'Ballantyne' syndrome, then the couple may elect to terminate the pregnancy.

In cases of CCAM, methods to predict the development of hydrops include the measurement of the CCAM volume using cystic adenomatoid volume ratio (CVR), described by the Philadelphia group.[34] The CVR may be useful in selecting fetuses at risk of developing hydrops and therefore organising increased fetal surveillance, with ultrasound and consideration for fetal intervention. Successful fetal therapy can be achieved using catheter shunt placement, as described in the section on fetal hydro-thorax. This form of fetal therapy is normally confined to fetuses where the CCAM has a large, predominant cyst and is not recommended in multicystic or predominantly solid CCAM lesions. Gestational age is also important, since it has been found that the insertion of a shunt at gestations less than 20 weeks can lead to increased risk of postnatal chest-wall abnormalities.

Other prenatal therapies may be worth consideration in fetuses with lung lesions. The simplest therapy is to administer a short course of maternal betamethasone, which may impair CCAM growth in some cases and can lead to amelioration of hydrops.[35] Open fetal surgery for specific cases has been successfully performed in two or three North American centres where highly specialised teams have developed the well-described procedures for fetal thoracotomy and resection of the lung mass. This type of treatment is not performed outside North America and is only considered if the couple have been extensively counselled by the multi-disciplinary team. In general terms, open fetal surgery is only performed in previable fetuses where hydrops has developed and there is no response to alternative fetal therapies or where it is considered that other strategies would be futile.

The final option for therapy in lung lesions is to consider the benefits of undertaking the tumour resection while the fetus or neonate remains on placental circulation. This is *ex utero* intrapartum treatment (the EXIT procedure) and merits separate description, since it may be useful for other fetal malformations, such as complex airway abnormalities, where a tracheostomy will be necessary immediately following delivery.

The EXIT procedure
An ex-utero intrapartum treatment (EXIT) delivery was initially described as offering benefit in the delivery of fetuses with complex lung lesions.[36] This is like performing a 'partial' caesarean section. Only the head and

neck and chest of the fetus or neonate are delivered. In situations where more extensive surgery is contemplated; for example, for resection of lung tumours the surgeon may need to use a uterine stapling device to minimise maternal bleeding from the uterine incision. The intrauterine volume can be maintained with the lower fetal body and continuous amnioinfusion of warmed Ringer lactate to prevent cord compression and hypothermia. Anaesthesia colleagues can maintain uterine relaxation by giving a high concentration of inhalational anaesthetic to preserve uteroplacental circulation.

EXIT has been adapted for use in the delivery of the fetus with a complex airway such as neck teratomas.[37] This involves a standard caesarean section operation, with the surgeon delivering only the head and neck. This allows adequate airway control while the fetus or neonate is maintained on placental bypass. Unfortunately this delivery strategy does not prevent a subset of neonatal deaths from ongoing respiratory factors.

Severe congenital heart disease

A small proportion of fetuses with congenital heart disease may benefit from *in utero* intervention. The aims of fetal therapy is to normalise circulatory imbalance in fetuses with stenosis or atresia of the aortic and pulmonary valves and defects associated with restriction or closure of the inter-atrial septum, such as transposition of the great arteries or hypoplastic left heart syndrome, where there is mitral and aortic atresia. Only a limited number of centres worldwide have performed these fetal interventions in a highly selected group of fetuses. The subject was reviewed by Gardiner in 2008.[38]

SACROCOCCYGEAL TERATOMA

Sacrococcygeal teratomas are the most common neoplasm in the fetus and newborn, with an estimated prevalence of 1/20 000 to 1/40 000 (Figure 5.17a). Female predominance is in the ratio of three to one. The blood supply to a sacrococcygeal teratoma commonly arises from the sacral artery. This vessel can enlarge to the size of the common iliac artery and can lead to vascular 'steal', causing high-output cardiac failure, placentomegaly, hydrops and ultimately fetal death. If the fetus is mature, caesarean delivery in a tertiary centre adjacent to paediatric surgical facilities should be performed. If hydrops develops before 28 weeks of gestation and the teratoma is amenable to resection, then fetal surgery could be considered. A retrospective review of 21 fetal sacrococcygeal teratomas diagnosed over 17 years (1980–97) reported a 19% *in utero* mortality rate and a 14% perinatal mortality rate.[39] Solid tumours had a particularly poor outcome. Developments in ultrafast fetal magnetic

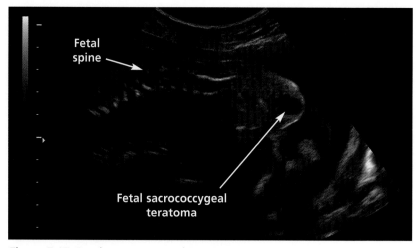

Figure 5.17 Fetal sacrococcygeal teratoma

resonance imaging (Figure 5.18) may improve the accuracy of antenatal diagnosis and aid counselling.

MYELOMENINGOCELE

Myelomeningocele (spina bifida) is one of the most common fetal malformations in the UK (Figure 5.19). It has a high rate of prenatal detection, owing to a combination of maternal serum AFP screening

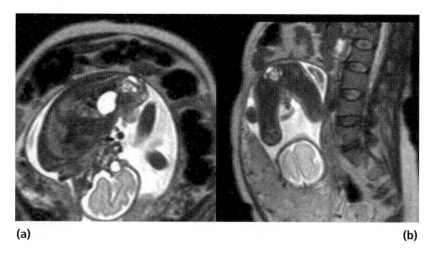

(a)　　　　　　　　　　　　　　　　　　　　(b)

Figure 5.18 Fetal MRI showing sacrococcygeal teratoma: (a) longitudinal; (b) transverse

programmes and because of the reliable cranial signs on routine fetal anomaly scanning.

The rationale for *in utero* repair of neural tube defects arises from experimental work in a fetal lamb model. This work demonstrated that the neurological deficit associated with open neural tube defects is not directly caused by the primary defect but rather is caused by chronic mechanical and chemical trauma when the unprotected neural tissue is exposed to the intrauterine environment. Thus, coverage of the myelomeningocele defect with skin flaps could be beneficial and this procedure has been performed at three centres in the USA. The largest series is that of the group at Vanderbilt University Medical Center, Nashville, Tennessee, who performed open fetal surgery on 29 cases of spina bifida.[40] This series showed that obstetric complications are low and neonatal outcome is improved, particularly a reduced incidence of ventriculoperitoneal shunting and almost complete disappearance of the Arnold–Chiari malformation in those fetuses undergoing fetal surgery, compared with a control group having conventional neonatal care. However, fetal surgery did not appear to improve bowel or bladder function and is associated with an increased incidence of premature delivery. There is currently a multicentre trial being conducted in the USA.[41]

Minimally invasive fetal surgery

In the 1970s, embryo fetoscopy was introduced as a diagnostic technique to obtain fetal blood for the diagnosis of haemoglobinopathies or to

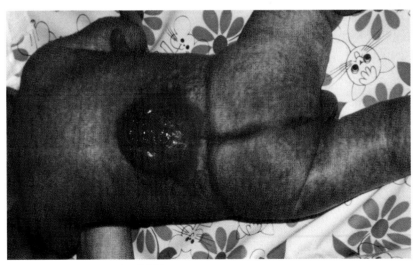

Figure 5.19 Open spina bifida

directly visualise malformations. The technique was abandoned in the 1980s because of advances in high-resolution ultrasound imaging. Developments in endoscopic equipment, especially with the introduction of small diameter fibrescopes, have increased the technical possibilities and reduced the invasiveness of endoscopy. Fetoscopy is now also being used to facilitate operations on the fetus and placenta and this will inevitably open up new opportunities to treat the fetus as a patient.

Key elements of the 'new fetoscopy' are the diameter, length field and angle of vision. Fibre endoscopes with diameters of 1.2–2.3 mm, working lengths of 25 cm and a 0-degree angle of view are used. A detailed description of the instrumentation used in fetoscopic surgery was published in 2009.[42] The endoscope can be introduced into the amniotic cavity through a sheath. To penetrate the maternal abdomen and uterine wall, the sheath is loaded with a sharp trocar and directed into place using real time ultrasound. The trocar is then withdrawn and the scope is passed. In addition, small instruments such as a laser fibre, forceps or scissors, as well as irrigation, can be used when required. The majority of fetoscopic procedures are performed percutaneously with local anaesthesia and without a formal cannula. However, in complex procedures like fetoscopic cord ligation or fetal surgery such as fetoscopic tracheal occlusion, multiple cannulae may be required.

FETOSCOPIC LASER ABLATION OF PLACENTAL VESSELS

Placental vascular communications exist in virtually all monochorionic pregnancies and only certain vascular patterns lead to the twin–twin transfusion syndrome (TTTS). TTTS appears to be based on the presence of one or a few arteriovenous anastomoses, in combination with a paucity of arterioarterious or venovenous anastomoses. The arterioarterious and venovenous anastomoses are found in abundance in uncomplicated monochorionic pregnancies. The arteriovenous anastomosis is not thought to be a true anatomical anastomosis but is considered by some researchers to be a cotyledon fed by an artery from one fetus and drained by a vein from the other twin.[43] The afferent and efferent branches of this shared cotyledon run over the placental surface and plunge into the chorionic plate almost at the same point. It is thought by some groups that identifying and ablating these vessels results in the elimination of the shared circulation and therefore in the resolution of the abnormal inter-twin blood transfer.

Neodymium: yttrium-aluminium-garnet (Nd:YAG) laser coagulation is usually performed under local or epidural anaesthesia with the use of a percutaneously inserted fetoscope. A 400–600 μm Nd:YAG laser fibre is introduced through the operative sheath. A combination of fetoscopic laser occlusion of chorioangiopagus vessels and systematic coagulation of all vessels crossing the inter-twin membrane is performed. The procedure also involves an amniodrainage procedure, as described earlier in this chapter.

FETOSCOPIC CORD OCCLUSION IN COMPLICATED MONOCHORIONIC TWINS

Fetoscopy has been used to assist selective termination by cord occlusion in cases of discordant monochorionic twins. The typical situation is that of the 'twin reversed arterial perfusion' (TRAP) sequence. In TRAP, the blood flows from the umbilical artery of the 'pump' twin in a reversed direction and via an arterioarterious anastomosis into the umbilical artery of the acardiac twin. This occurs in approximately 1% of monochorionic twins and can lead to a situation of high-output cardiac failure in the pump twin. This situation has an extremely poor prognosis and therefore prophylactic intervention when the acardiac–pump twin ratio exceeds 50%[44] and urgent intervention when the ratio is greater than 70%.[45]

Other complications of monochorionic twins that may be amenable to cord occlusion include the presence of a major anomaly in one twin, particularly of the central nervous system, and other conditions with a poor prognosis. In such circumstances, conventional techniques for feticide with intracardiac injection of potassium chloride cannot be carried out in view of the shared circulations and hence the likelihood of fetal death of the unaffected co-twin.

Other procedures have been developed to occlude umbilical blood flow to the affected twin instantly and permanently. These techniques include:

- ultrasound-guided sclerosation or embolisation of major fetal vessels using agents such as absolute alcohol, thrombogenic coils or enbucrilate gel[46]
- Nd:YAG laser for cord coagulation[47]
- surgical ligation of the cord under either fetoscopic or ultrasound guidance[47]
- bipolar coagulation of the umbilical cord under ultrasound guidance[48,49]
- monopolar thermocoagulation under ultrasound guidance[44]
- radiofrequency ablation.[50]

The success rate for absolute alcohol or enbucrilate gel instillation is only 30% and this technique should therefore now be discouraged. The problem with surgical cord ligation either under fetoscopic or ultrasound guidance is that there is a relatively high rate of PPROM (30%). The preferred procedure for cord ablation is either mono- or bipolar coagulation under ultrasound guidance and this technique can be performed in most fetal medicine units.

Radiofrequency ablation is a promising new technique for selective reduction in TRAP sequence and multifetal pregnancy reduction in monochorionic twins. The preliminary results are encouraging, with one series reporting an 86% survival rate and a low risk of PPROM.[51]

COMPLICATIONS OF OPERATIVE FETOSCOPY

The most important adverse effect of operative fetoscopy is the high risk of PPROM. Even after the 'learning curve' of the procedure, the incidence of iatrogenic PPROM remains significant. Other complications are the same as those with serial amnioreductions, such as chorioamnionitis and placental abruption. Since the 'new fetoscopy' is a new method of fetal therapy, it is vital that prospective audit of the fetoscopic techniques performed in fetal medicine centres takes place. A registry of such fetoscopic procedures performed worldwide has now been established whose primary objective is to establish accurate data on maternal and fetal safety that can be used in counselling prospective parents.[52]

Fetal pain and awareness

In light of the current availability of fetal treatment options, there has been considerable ethical and scientific debate concerning fetal pain and awareness. This resulted in the RCOG establishing an initial working party and making recommendations.[53] The initial conclusions were that there is some evidence of fetal awareness above 22 weeks of gestation and the working party recommended that, should invasive fetal procedures be performed at this gestation or above, they should be carried out only after maternal and/or fetal analgesia was administered. However, a RCOG working party established to review this evidence has concluded that there is little evidence for fetal pain and awareness above 22 weeks of gestation and current recommendations are that fetal analgesia is not required.[54] However there is still benefit in providing some sedation to the mother undergoing invasive procedures at later gestations.[54] This can be given in the form of maternal sedation with opiates before the procedure commences.

Future therapies

STEM CELL TRANSPLANTATION

Bone marrow transplantation can be used to treat many severe congenital and acquired haematological disorders. However, a large number of patients have no compatible donors and this can lead to rejection, in the form of graft-versus-host disease, which is induced by T lymphocytes. In view of the natural lack of T cells during early development, fetal liver stem cells can reconstitute the haematopoietic and lymphopoietic systems without producing graft-versus-host disease. In view of this, stem cell transplantation *in utero* has been successfully performed using fetal liver cells during early human fetal development following prenatal diagnosis. The main indications for fetal stem cell transplantation are:

- chronic granulomatous disease
- severe combined immunodeficiency
- β-thalassaemia
- sickle cell disease
- a fetus which will have neonatal organ failure and can be made immune tolerant.

The advantages of stem cell transplantation over postnatal therapy are shown in Box 5.2. *In utero* transplantation has been successfully performed in a handful of cases in specialised centres and may offer a promising potential new fetal therapy for the severely sick fetus. The subject is well described by several authors.[55,56]

GENE THERAPY

As the Human Genome Project attempts to map our estimated 50 000–200 000 genes, much is already known about the structure of many genes and the mutations which cause disease states. The ultimate goal is to progress from this knowledge to attempting to cure genetic disease by gene therapy. The main areas of research involve identifying the best approaches for gene transfer and whether these should be using physical methods such as direct DNA injection, by liposome fusion or by biological vectors using retro or adenoviruses. Some of the selected disease models that are currently being studied are:

- defects in haematopoietic cell function
- haemophilia
- familial hypercholesterolaemia

- growth deficiency
- cancer
- cystic fibrosis
- muscle gene therapy.

The major issues that remain unresolved are the length of time for which interventions will provide the desired therapeutic effect and whether expression of the transferred gene will really give clinical benefit. As well as aiding in the treatment of genetic diseases, it is likely that gene therapy will have benefit for other conditions that lead to morbidity and in which transfection (the process of infecting cells with purified DNA or RNA isolated from a virus after a specific pretreatment) of the fetus is more efficient than postnatal therapy. Currently, gene therapy remains an experimental procedure. This evolving subject is covered elsewhere.[57,58]

Ethics of fetal therapy

The pregnant woman is under no obligation to confer the status of being a patient on her previable fetus simply because there exists a fetal therapy. The same is true for fetal therapy on the viable fetus, who is properly judged to be a patient. Fetal therapy should be considered when that intervention would benefit the fetus and the risks of the treatment are acceptable to the pregnant woman. McCullough and Chervenak consider that three criteria should be satisfied:[59]

- when invasive therapy of the viable fetus is reliably judged to have a very high probability of being life saving or of preventing serious or irreversible disease, injury, or handicap for the fetus and for the child that the fetus can become.
- when such therapy is reliably judged to involve low mortality risk and low or manageable risk of serious disease, injury or handicap to the viable fetus and the child it can become.
- when the mortality risk to the pregnant woman is reliably judged to be very low and when the risk of disease, injury or handicap to the pregnant woman is reliably judged to be low or manageable.

Such decision making is complex but the obligations owed to the pregnant woman and to the fetal patient as outlined are mandatory and, as this new branch of perinatal medicine grows, it will be essential to apply such ethical considerations to many more areas of fetal therapy. The ethics of fetal therapy are described in detail by Noble and Rodeck.[60]

References

1. National Collaborating Centre for Women's and Children's Health. *Antenatal Care: Routine Care for the Healthy Pregnant Women*. 2nd ed. London: RCOG Press; 2008 [http://guidance.nice.org.uk/CG62]. p. 134–52.

2. Little J, Ellwood M. Geographical variation. In: Ellwood JM, Little J, Ellwood JH. *The Epidemiology and Control of Neural Tube Defects*. Oxford: Oxford University Press; 1992. p. 96–145.

3. Richmond S, Atkins J. A population-based study of the prenatal diagnosis of congenital malformation over 16 years. *BJOG* 2005;112:1349–57.

4. Medical Research Council Vitamin Study Research Group. Prevention of neural tube defects: results of the Medical Research Council Vitamin Study Research Group. *Lancet* 1991;338:131–7.

5. Forest MG, David M. [Prevention of sexual ambiguity in children with 21-hydroxylase deficiency by treatment in utero.] *Pediatrie* 1992;47;351–7 [French].

6. Rijnders RJ, van der Schoot CE, Bossers B, de Vroede MA, Christianes GC. Fetal sex determination from maternal plasma in pregnancies at risk for congenital adrenal hyperplasia. *Obstet Gynecol* 2001;98:374–8.

7. Api O, Carvalho J. Fetal dysrhythmias. *Best Pract Res Clin Obstet Gynaecol* 2008;22(1):31–48.

8. Blanch G, Walkinshaw SA, Walsh K. Cardioversion of fetal tachyarrythmias with adenosine. *Lancet* 1994;344:1646.

9. Simpson JM. Fetal arrythmias. In: Allan L, Hornberger L, Sharland G, editors. *Textbook of Fetal Cardiology*. London: Greenwich Medical Media; 2000. p. 421–7.

10. Jaeggi ET, Fouron JC, Silverman ED, Ryan G, Smallhorn J, Hornberger LK. Transplacental fetal treatment improves the outcome of prenatally diagnosed complete atrioventricular block without structural heart disease. *Circulation* 2004;110:1542–8.

11. Daniels G, Finning K, Soothill P. Fetal blood group genotyping from DNA from maternal plasma: an important advance in the management of the prevention of haemolytic disease of the fetus and newborn. *Vox Sang* 2004;87:225–32.

12. Moise KJ. Red blood cell alloimmunisation in pregnancy. *Semin Haematol* 2005;42:169–78.

13. Mari G, Deter RL, Carpenter RL, Rahman F, Zimmerman R, Moise KJ Jr, *et al*. Noninvasive diagnosis by Doppler ultrasonography of fetal anaemia due to maternal red-cell alloimmunization. Collaborative group for Doppler assessmentof the blood velocity in anemic fetuses. *N Eng J Med* 2000;342:9–14.

14. Oepkes D, Seaward PG, Vandenbussche FP, Windrim R, Kingdom J, Beyene J, *et al*. Doppler ultrasonography versus amniocentesis to predict fetal anaemia. *N Engl J Med* 2006;355:156–64.

15. Brennand J, Cameron AD. Fetal anaemia; diagnosis and management. *Best Pract Res Clin Obstet Gynaecol* 2008;22(1):15–29.

16. Van Kamp IL, Klumper FJ, Oepkes D, Meerman RH, Scherjon SA, Vandenbussche FP, *et al*. Complications of intrauterine intravascular transfusion for fetal anaemia due to maternal red-cell alloimmunization. *Am J Obstet Gynecol* 2005;192:171–7.

17. Bussel JB; Neonatal Immune Thrombocytopenia Study Group. Neonatal alloimmune thrombocytopenia (NAIT): information derived from a prospective international registry. *Paediatr Res* 1988;23:337.

18. Mackenzie FM, Brennand J, Peterkin M, Cameron AD. Management of fetal alloimmune thrombocytopenia: a less invasive option? *J Obstet Gynecol* 1999;19:119–21.

19. Van den Akker ESA, Oepkes D. Fetal and neonatal alloimmune thrombocytopenia. *Best Pract Res Clin Obstet Gynaecol* 2008;22:3–14.

20. Morris RK, Quinlan- Jones E, Kilby M, Khan KS. Systematic review of accuracy of fetal urine analysis to predict poor postnatal renal function in cases of congenital urinary tract obstruction. *Prenat Diagn* 2007;27:900–11.

21. Freedman AL, Johnson MP, Smith CA, Gonzalez R, Evans MI. Long-term outcome in children after antenatal intervention for obstructive uropathies. *Lancet* 1999;354:374–7.

22. Morris RK, Malin GL,Khan KS Kilby. Systematic review of the effectiveness of antenatal intervention for the treatment of congenital lower urinary tract obstruction. *BJOG* 2010;117:382–90.

23. National Institute for Health and Clinical Excellence. *Fetal Vesico Amniotic Shunt for Lower Urinary Tract Obstruction*. NICE Interventional Procedure Guidance. London: NICE; 2006.

24. Morris RK, Kilby MD. Congenital urinary tract obstruction. *Best Pract Res Clin Obstet Gynaecol* 2008;22(1): 97–122.

25. Yinon Y, Kelly E, Ryan G. Fetal pleural effusions. *Best Pract Res Clin Obstet Gynaecol* 2008;22(1):77–96.

26. Knox EM, Kilby MD, Martin WL Khan KS. In utero pulmonary drainage in the management of primary hydrothorax and congenital cystic lung lesion: a systematic review. *Ultrasound Obstet Gynecol* 2006;28:726–34.

27. Chen M, Shih JC, Wang BT, Chen CP, Yu CL. Fetal OK-432 pleurodesis: complete or incomplete? *Ultrasound Obstet Gynecol* 2005;26:791–3.

28. Fisk NM, Ronderos-Dumit D, Soliani A, Nicolini U, Vaughan J, Rodeck CH. Diagnostic and therapeutic transabdominal amnioinfusion in oligohydramnios. *Obstet Gynecol* 1991;78:270–8.

29. Gucciardo L, Deprest J, Done' E, Van Mieghem T, Van de Velde M, Gratacos E, *et al*. Prediction of outcome in isolated congenital diaphragmatic hernia and its consequences for fetal therapy. *Best Pract Res Clin Obstet Gynaecol* 2008;22(1):123–38.

30. Jani J, Nicolaides KH, Keller RL, Benachi A, Peralta CF, Favre R, *et al*. Observed to expected lung area to head circumference ratio in the prediction of survival in fetuses with isolated diaphragmatic hernia. *Ultrasound Obstet Gynecol* 2007;30:67–71.

31. Harrison MR, Keller RL, Hawgood SB, Kitterman JA, Sandberg PL, Farmer DL, *et al*. A randomized trial of fetal endoscopic tracheal occlusion for severe congenital diaphragmatic hernia. *N Engl J Med* 2003;349:1916–24.

32. Deprest J, Gratacos E, Nicolaides KH; FETO Task Group. Fetoscopic tracheal occlusion (FETO) for severe congenital diaphragmatic hernia: evolution of a technique and preliminary results. *Ultrasound Obstet Gynecol* 2004;24:121–6.

33. Adzick NS, Harrison MR, Crombleholme TM, Flake AW, Howell LJ. Fetal lung lesions: management and outcome. *Am J Obstet Gynecol* 1998;179:884–9.

34. Crombleholme TM, Coleman B, Hedrick H, Liechty K, Howell L, Flake AW, *et al*. Cystic adenomatoid malformation volume ratio predicts outcome in prenatally diagnosed cystic adenomatoid malformation of the lung. *J Pediatr Surg* 2002;37:331–8.

35. Peranteau WH, Wilson RD, Liechty KW, Johnson MP, Bebbington MW, Hedrick HL, *et al*. The effect of maternal betamethasone administration on prenatal congenital cystic adenomatoid malformation growth and fetal survival. *Fetal Diagn Ther* 2007;22:365–71.

36. Hedrick HL, Flake AW, Crombleholme TM, Howell LJ, Johnson MP, Wilson RD, *et al*. The ex utero intrapartum (EXIT) procedure for high risk lung lesions. *J Pediatr Surg* 2005;40:1038–43.

37. McDevitt H, Kubba H, Macara L, Reynolds B, Simpson J. Four cases of congenital airway obstruction: optimising perinatal management. *Acta Paediatr* 2007;96:1542–5.

38. Gardiner HM. In utero intervention for severe congenital heart disease. *Best Pract Res Clin Obstet Gynaecol* 2008;22(1):49–61.

39. Holterman AX, Filiatrault D, Lallier M, Youssef S. The natural history of sacrococcygeal teratomas diagnosed through routine obstetric sonogram: a single institution experience. *J Paediatr Surg* 1998;33:899–903.

40. Bruner JP, Tulipan N, Paschall RL, Boehm FH, Walsh WF, Silva SR, *et al*. Fetal surgery for myelomeningocoele and the incidence of shunt dependent hydrocephalus. *JAMA* 1999;282:1819–25.

41. Eunice Kennedy Shriver National Institute of Child Health and Human Development. MOMS: Management of Myelomeningocele Study [www.spinabifidamoms.com]. Trial registration [http://clinicaltrials.gov/ct2/show/NCT00060606].

42. Klaritsch P, Albert K, Van Mieghem T, Gucciardo L, Done E, Bynens B, *et al*. Instrumental requirements for minimally invasive fetal surgery. *BJOG* 2009;116:188–97.

43. Van Gemert MJ, Major AL, Scherjon SA. Placental anatomy, fetal demise and therapeutic intervention in monochorionic twins and the transfusion syndrome: new hypothesis. *Eur J Obstet Gynecol* 1998;78:53–62.

44. Tan TY, Sepulveda W. Acardiac twin: a systematic review of minimally invasive treatment modalities. *Ultrasound Obstet Gynecol* 2003;22:409–19.

45. Weisz B, Peltz, Chayen B, Oren M, Zalel Y, Achiron R, *et al*. Tailored management of twin reversed arterial perfusion (TRAP) sequence. *Ultrasound Obstet Gynecol* 2004;23:451–5.

46. Denbow ML, Overton TG, Duncan KR, Cox PM, Fisk NM. High failure rate of umbilical vessel occlusion by ultrasound guided injection of absolute alcohol or enbucrilate gel. *Prenat Diagn* 1999;19:527–32.

47. Deprest JA, Van Ballaer PP, Evrard VA, Peers KH, Spitz B, Steegers EA, *et al*. Experience with fetoscopic cord ligation. *Eur J Obstet Gynecol Reprod Biol* 1998;81:157–64.

48. Lewi L, Gratacos E, Ortibus E, Van Schoubroeck D, Carreras E, Higueras T, *et al.* Pregnancy and infant outcome of 80 consecutive cord coagulations in complicated monochorionic multiple pregnancies. *Am J Obstet Gynecol* 2006;194:782–9.

49. Deprest JA, Audibert F, Van Schoubroeck D, Hecher K, Mahieu-Caputo D. Bipolar cord coagulation of the umbilical cord in complicated monochorionic twin pregnancy. *Am J Obstet Gynecol* 2000;182:340–5.

50. Wong AE, Sepulveda W. Acardiac anomaly: current issues in prenatal assessment and treatment. *Prenat Diagn* 2005;25:796–806.

51. Lee H, Wagner AJ, Sy E, Ball R, Feldstein VA, Goldstein RB, *et al.* Efficacy of radiofrequency ablation for twin reversed arterial perfusion sequence. *Am J Obstet Gynecol* 2007;196:459–64.

52. Eurofetus Programme. Endoscopic access to the fetoplacental unit: from experimental to clinical applications [www.Eurofetus.org].

53. Royal College of Obstetricians and Gynaecologists. *Fetal Awareness: Report of a Working Party*. London: RCOG; 1997.

54. Royal College of Obstetricians and Gynaecologists. *Fetal Awareness: Review of Research and Recommendations for Practice. Report of a Working Party*. London: RCOG; 2010 [www.rcog.org.uk/fetal-awareness-reviews-research-and-recommendations-practice].

55. Tiblad E, Westgren M. Fetal stem cell transplantation. *Best Pract Res Clin Obstet Gynecol* 2008;22(1):189–201.

56. Scherjon S, Anker E. In utero stem cell transplantation. In: Rodeck CH, Whittle MJ, editors. *Fetal Medicine: Basic Science and Clinical Practice*. 2nd ed. London: Churchill Livingstone; 2009. p. 678–88.

57. David AL, Peebles D. Gene therapy for the fetus: is there a future? *Best Pract Res Clin Obstet Gynecol* 2008;22(1):203–18.

58. David A, Rodeck CH. Fetal gene therapy. In: Rodeck CH, Whittle MJ, editors. *Fetal Medicine: Basic Science and Clinical Practice*. 2nd ed. London: Churchill Livingstone; 2009. p. 689–99.

59. McCullough LB, Chervenak FA. *Ethics in Obstetrics and Gynaecology*. New York: Oxford University Press; 1994.

60. Noble R, Rodeck CH. Ethical considerations of fetal therapy. *Best Pract Res Clin Obstet Gynecol* 2008;22(1):219–31.

6 Prenatal diagnosis and management of non-immune hydrops fetalis

Introduction

Non-immune hydrops fetalis (NIHF) is an uncommon but important condition accounting for a disproportionate 3% of overall perinatal mortality (Figure 6.1). With the decline in rhesus isoimmunisation, non-immunological causes have become responsible for the majority of fetal hydrops. Ballantyne was first to report that NIHF represents an 'end-stage condition' of different disease processes in 1892.[1] The variety of conditions that cause or are associated with fetal hydrops makes it a challenge for the obstetrician to find the cause and decide on the management of this pregnancy complication in order to reduce the high perinatal loss. With the increasing use of ultrasound, prenatal diagnosis is possible at an earlier gestational age.

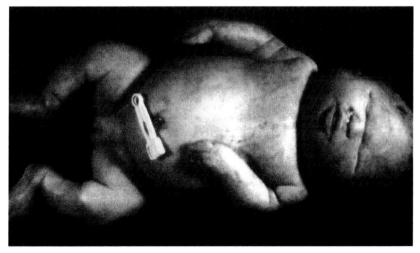

Figure 6.1 Stillborn hydropic neonate

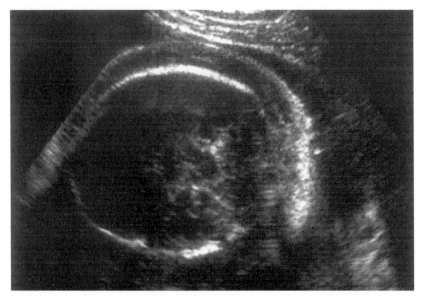

Figure 6.2 Scalp oedema: 'halo' sign

NIHF is defined as generalised oedema of soft tissues irrespective of the presence of effusions or placental oedema without evidence of isoimmunisation (Figures 6.2, 6.3). It is reported to occur in between 1/1500 and

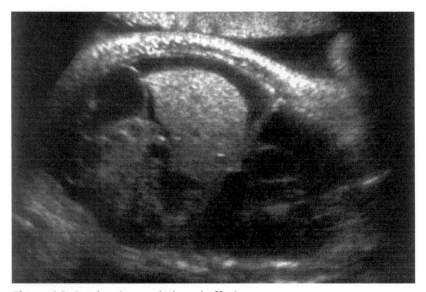

Figure 6.3 Fetal ascites and pleural effusions

1/4000 pregnancies. However, one series would suggest that the current incidence might be as high as one in 800 pregnancies.[2]

It is important to develop a logical sequence for the investigation and obstetric management of NIHF. It is recommended to proceed from the least invasive evaluation methods (serum studies, ultrasound, echo-cardiography) to the more invasive and sophisticated methods (chorionic villus sampling and cordocentesis) and thus it is likely that referral to a fetal medicine department will be required (Box 6.1).

BOX 6.1 PROTOCOL FOR THE INVESTIGATION AND MANAGEMENT OF NON-IMMUNE HYDROPS (SWAIN *et al.* 1999)[2]

History

1 Age, parity, gestation
2 Previous scan findings in this pregnancy
3 Past medical and obstetric history
4 Family history (e.g. metabolic disorders)
5 Recent infections and contacts
6 Reason for referral

Maternal investigations

1 Full blood count
2 Blood group and antibodies
3 Haemoglobin electrophoresis (-thalassaemia carriers)
4 Kleihauer–Betke test (fetomaternal haemorrhage)
5 Infection screening for toxoplasma, cytomegalovirus, rubella, parvovirus, syphilis, serology
6 Autoantibody screen (systemic lupus erythematosus, Anti Ro and La)
7 Oral glucose tolerance test

Fetal investigations

1 Detailed abnormality scan including fetal echocardiography
2 Amniotic fluid index
3 Placental morphology and thickness
4 Doppler flow velocity studies of:
       umbilical artery
       middle cerebral artery
       tricuspid ejection velocity
5 M-mode study of the heart:
       cardiac biometry
       heart rate and rhythm

(continued on following page)

To improve survival, early diagnosis must be made prenatally. Ultrasound is the single most useful tool not only in the prenatal diagnostic evaluation but also in the assessment of the disease progression in a fetus with NIHF.

Aetiology

The major causes of NIHF are chromosomal abnormality, structural cardiovascular disease, cardiac dysrhythmias, abnormalities of the fetal thorax, haematological disorders and infections. A cause is established in more than 50% of cases, with no explanation being found in 13–35%. There is an inverse relationship between the incidence of karyotype abnormalities and gestation at presentation and it is unusual not to find a cause in early NIHF.

Specific causes

CHROMOSOMAL ABNORMALITIES

Studies from Australia have shown that 52% of cases before 20 weeks of gestation have a karyotypic anomaly, whereas 28% at gestations over 20 weeks have a chromosomal abnormality. The most frequently found abnormalities are trisomy 21 and Turner syndrome, although trisomies 13,

16, 18 and triploidy are not infrequent. Women whose fetus has sonographic appearances suggestive of hydrops should be offered fetal karyotyping using the most appropriate method.[3] This should include a long-term culture, since a small proportion of NIHF fetuses have rarer chromosomal rearrangements.

CARDIOVASCULAR DISEASE

The combination of anatomical cardiac disease and fetal dysrhythmias makes cardiovascular disease the second most common group of causes. Approximately 25% of cases of NIHF have an underlying cardiac or vascular abnormality. Many of the structural defects also have karyotypic abnormality. Anomalies that lead to increased right-sided atrial pressure are the most likely to lead to NIHF. The lesions with significant left-sided obstruction are the most common, as they result in increased right ventricular flow. Premature closure of the foramen ovale or ductus arteriosus and Ebstein's anomaly also lead to NIHF. Hydrops has also been found with septal defects, transposition of the great arteries, Fallot's tetralogy and truncus arteriosus.

Fetal cardiac dysrhythmias in the form of either tachy- or bradycardias can also lead to NIHF. Tachydysrhythmias are the most common, with

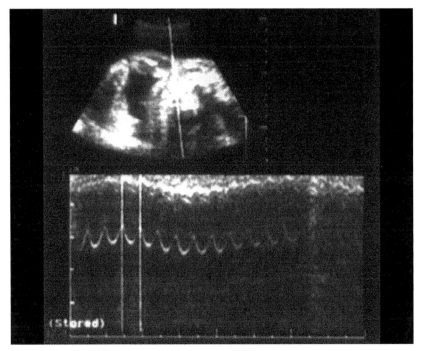

Figure 6.4 Fetal supraventricular tachycardia

supraventricular tachycardia being the cause of 50% of cases (Figure 6.4). Atrioventricular re-entrant tachycardias are the next most frequent and these are followed by atrial flutter. Fetal bradycardias, including congenital complete fetal heart block, are also associated with NIHF. Bradycardias may be associated with either structural congenital heart disease or with maternal connective disorder.[4]

Fetal echocardiography may be indicated if a major cardiac defect is suspected. Recognition of fetal cardiac arrhythmias in the absence of structural cardiac defect offers the opportunity for therapeutic intervention, in the form of maternal medication combined with continued observation and planned delivery. This is discussed in more detail in Chapter 5.

Rarer cardiovascular causes of NIHF include fetal or placental arteriovenous shunts that cause vascular steal and hyperdynamic circulation, such as sacrococcygeal teratoma and vein of Galen aneurysm. Placental tumours, such as chorioangioma, can also lead to NIHF and so a through ultrasound examination of both fetus and placenta is imperative in cases of NIHF.

ABNORMALITIES OF THE FETAL THORAX

Any space-occupying lesion in the chest can lead to NIHF. The most common causes are congenital cystic adenomatoid malformation of the lung (CCAM), congenital diaphragmatic hernia, pulmonary sequestration and isolated hydrothorax, including chylothorax. The combination of these pathologies with NIHF leads to a poor prognosis in a large percentage of cases. This has led fetal medicine specialists and paediatric surgeons to explore fetal treatment options, including open resection of CCAM during fetal life. Drainage procedures using ultrasound-guided techniques have also been performed in CCAM and in cases of hydrothorax with mixed results. This exciting new area is considered in more detail in Chapter 5.

SKELETAL DYSPLASIAS

Approximately 2–5% of cases of NIHF are caused by skeletal dysplasia, mainly in those syndromes that have associated severe thoracic restriction, such as thanatophoric dwarfism and Jeune syndrome (asphyxiating thoracic dysplasia).

FETAL AKINESIA SYNDROMES

Fetal akinesia syndromes account for a similar proportion of NIHF as the skeletal dysplasias. They include Pena–Shokeir syndrome, myotonic dystrophy, Neu Laxova syndrome and arthrogryposis multiplex. Most are lethal in the neonatal period and have an autosomal recessive inheritance apart from myotonic dystrophy, which is autosomal dominant.

OTHER GENETIC CAUSES

A large number of genetic diseases can present as NIHF. It is estimated that 10–15% of all NIHF is caused by genetic diseases that can be grouped into metabolic disorders, such as the mucopolysaccharidoses, and multiple malformation syndromes, such as Noonan and Cornelia de Lange syndromes. These are important diagnoses to establish, since they have a high (one in four) risk of recurrence.

Investigation of non-infectious NIHF

Investigation should begin with a detailed maternal history, following which is the key investigation, a detailed high-resolution ultrasound scan of the pregnancy. Examination of the fetal anatomy, including fetal echocardiography, should be performed by an experienced ultrasonographer. This may require referral to a fetal medicine centre. If no obvious structural abnormality is seen, the mother should have further counselling and be offered invasive fetal testing. Chorionic villus sampling should be recommended for those women with diagnosis of NIHF in the late first trimester or early second trimester. In some cases, amniocentesis may be preferred, since it allows sampling for viral or bacterial culture and metabolic testing. Liquor should be stored for future testing in those cases where the aetiology is unclear. In later gestations (over 20 weeks), fetal blood sampling by cordocentesis is the preferred invasive test. This is particularly the case if there is a suspicion of fetal anaemia from middle cerebral artery Doppler studies. This allows a rapid diagnosis of chromosomal and metabolic disorders. Couples should have in-depth counselling and, in particular, it should be explained that the risk of complications with cordocentesis is higher in cases of NIHF. Surviving neonates should have extensive investigations, encompassing a multidisciplinary approach involving medical geneticists and paediatric metabolic medicine specialists, in an attempt to obtain a diagnosis. In cases of perinatal loss, a full postmortem examination, including histology, should be carried out. In addition, radiology and genetics input may help. Storage of fetal and placental DNA for future studies should go ahead only after full written consent is obtained.

Management of non-infectious NIHF

Despite the availability of fetal therapy, for some cases of NIHF, the overall prognosis for this condition remains poor. Occasionally, the maternal mirror or Ballantyne syndrome will develop. This leads to severe oedema, proteinuria and hypertension in the mothers of fetuses with NIHF, with these symptoms resolving if the fetal hydrops resolves.[5]

In those cases diagnosed early that have such a poor outlook, termination of pregnancy should be discussed. This approach should also be taken when serious associated underlying pathology is also present. The situation of early planned preterm birth should also be avoided, since this leads to further morbidity and mortality for the neonate.

Fetal therapy in the form of pleuroamniotic shunting has been successfully attempted in cases where the predominant finding is of pleural effusions but not in the cases of gross fetal ascites with peritoneoamniotic shunting. Other proposed pharmacological treatments have been the use of maternal steroids in cases of complete heart block and digoxin and other antiarrhythmic agents in cardiac dysrhythmias. Some success has also been reported with the use of digoxin and aggressive amnioreduction in cases with non-cardiac cause of NIHF.

Fetal infection

Infectious causes contribute approximately 5% of cases with NIHF. The specific issues concerning parvovirus are discussed in Chapter 10.

Fetal anaemia

Fetal anaemia is one of the most common causes of NIHF, especially if infection by human parvovirus B19 is included. Other haematological causes include α-thalassaemia and glucose-6-phosphate dehydrogenase deficiency. Fetomaternal haemorrhage is also associated with fetal anaemia and NIHF. Some of the fetal anaemias, such as those caused by parvovirus, can be treated with intrauterine transfusions, as discussed in Chapter 5.

Conclusion

NIHF represents a wide spectrum of fetal disease. Many of the aetiologies are associated with an extremely poor outcome. A systematic process of investigation for the underlying cause of hydrops will reveal the cause in the majority (80%) of cases. The diagnosis, investigation and management of NIHF remains both an academic and clinical challenge that should be actively pursued using a multidisciplinary approach in the years ahead.

References

1. Ballantyne JW. *The Diseases and Deformities of the Fetus*. Edinburgh: Oliver and Boyd; 1892.
2. Swain S, Cameron A, McNay M, Howatson AG. Prenatal diagnosis and management of nonimmune hydrops fetalis. *Aust N Z J Obstet Gynaecol* 1999;39:285–90.

3. Cameron AD, Murphy KW, McNay MB, Mathers AM, Kingdom J, Aitken JA, *et al*. Midtrimester chorionic villus sampling; an alternative approach? *Am J Obstet Gynecol* 1994;171:1035–7.

4. Jaeggi ET, Hornberger LK, Smallhorn JF, Fouron JC. Prenatal Diagnosis of complete atrioventricular block associated with structural heart disease: combined experience of two tertiary centres and review of the literature. *Ultrasound Obstet Gynecol* 2005;26:16–21.

5. Duthie SJ, Walkinshaw SA. Parvovirus associated fetal hydrops: reversal of pregnancy induced proteinuric hypertension by in utero fetal transfusion. *Br J Obstet Gynaecol* 1995;102:1011–13.

Further reading

Hyett J. Fetal hydrops. In: *Fetal Medicine: Basic Science and Clinical Practice*. Rodeck CH, Whittle MJ, editors. London: Churchill Livingstone; 2008.

7 Termination of pregnancy for fetal abnormality

Introduction

The United Kingdom Abortion Act was passed in 1967 and amended in 1990 when the Human Fertilisation and Embryology Act was passed. The main changes were that an upper time limit of 24 weeks was introduced for the termination of pregnancy where fetal abnormality was not the indication for the procedure. There was also the removal of any time limit if a termination was being carried out for fetal abnormality, such that no offence was committed under either the law relating to abortion or the Infant Life Preservation Act 1929 if a medical practitioner was involved within the clauses of the Abortion Act in this work.

The main clause concerning termination for fetal abnormality is found in Section I(d) of the Act and this states that termination is permitted when two registered medical practitioners are of an opinion formed in good faith that 'there is substantial risk that if the child were born it would suffer from such physical or mental abnormalities as to be seriously handicapped'.

This, therefore, forms the basis of legal termination of pregnancy for fetal abnormality in the UK. The stage of pregnancy at which the diagnosis is made and the time of pregnancy when the decision to perform a termination is made are crucial in terms of how the procedure may be performed. The decision to terminate a pregnancy because of fetal abnormality is often extremely difficult and it is vital that a comprehensive counselling service is available to the couple concerned before undertaking the procedure. This should involve multidisciplinary teamwork from obstetricians, midwives, geneticists and paediatricians, where appropriate. This complex area is dealt with in detail by Fisher and Staham.[1]

First trimester of pregnancy

The majority of fetal malformations detected in the first trimester are diagnosed between 10 and 14 weeks of gestation. At this stage of pregnancy, the method of choice for termination is vacuum aspiration. Although abortion can be induced by antigestagens and prostaglandins, the incidence of incomplete abortion is high and many women require surgical evacuation of the uterus. When performing suction termination, the cervix should be pre-treated using a prostaglandin analogue, such as gemeprost 1 mg vaginally or the prostaglandin E_1 analogue misoprostol 400 micrograms (two 200-microgram tablets) vaginally. Both these cervical ripening agents need to be administered 3 hours before surgery for maximum benefit.

Although vacuum aspiration is an extremely safe operation, rates of blood loss and other complications rise as gestation advances. Haemorrhage at the time of abortion is rare, complicating around 1.5/1000 abortions overall. The rate is lower for early abortions (1.2/1000 at less than 13 weeks and 8.5/1000 at over 20 weeks). Uterine perforation at the time of surgical abortion is rare. The incidence is approximately 1.4/1000, with the rate being lower early in pregnancy and when performed by experienced clinicians. This is also the case with cervical trauma, which occurs in less than 1% of cases. Genital tract infection of varying degrees of severity occurs in up to 10% of cases. This can be reduced by administering periabortion antibiotic prophylaxis using the regimens described in the RCOG Guideline.[2] It is important, therefore, to refer the woman for abortion promptly after the decision to terminate the pregnancy has been made.

Mid-trimester abortion

It is possible to induce abortion at this stage of pregnancy either medically or surgically. Surgical dilatation and evacuation (D&E) is the method of choice in the USA but in the UK its use is confined largely to gynaecologists in private practice. It may be necessary to dilate the cervix up to a diameter of 20 mm before the fetal parts can be extracted. Historically, it has been considered that D&E is a risk factor for subsequent adverse pregnancy outcomes, including cervical weakness, pregnancy loss and preterm birth. A retrospective case series which included 600 women who underwent mid-trimester D&E between 1996 and 2000 found that rates of adverse pregnancy outcomes appeared similar to those of unselected populations. The authors concluded that 'second-trimester D&E is not a risk factor for mid-trimester pregnancy loss or spontaneous preterm birth'.[3]

The alternative medical methods involve inducing uterine contractions so that the fetus is expelled from the uterus. In the past, a variety of substances, such as hypertonic saline and urea, together with prostaglandin, were either injected directly into the amniotic sac or instilled through the cervix into the extra-amniotic space using a Foley catheter connected to a pump. These methods were relatively inefficient and labour was prolonged, in some cases for more than 48 hours and so carried a substantial increase in the risk of infection. There was also the risk of cardiovascular collapse from inadvertent injection of prostaglandin or hypertonic solution directly into the bloodstream. Instillation has largely been replaced by vaginal prostaglandins in combination with mifepristone pretreatment.

It is well established that the administration of mifepristone (a progesterone antagonist) 36–48 hours before induction of abortion with prostaglandins will significantly reduce the induction-to-abortion interval. Therefore, women should be given the option of this treatment. The recommended dosage regimens are described in detail in the RCOG Guideline.[2]

It is the responsibility of the doctor prescribing mifepristone to make sure that there are no contraindications to treatment with this drug. Once administered, the woman should remain in hospital for up to 1 hour to ensure that there are no adverse effects (occasionally nausea and vomiting). She can then go home to be readmitted 36–48 hours later.

On admission, a full blood count, group and save are taken. A cannula should be sited but there is no need to commence intravenous fluids immediately. Abortion is induced with the prostaglandin E_1 analogue, misoprostol. Alternatively, the other analogue, gemeprost 1 mg, can be given. This is administered vaginally. With misoprostol, the first dose is 800 micrograms vaginally followed by 400-microgram doses orally on a 3-hourly basis, to a maximum of five doses in total. For gemeprost, the dose is 1 mg repeated at intervals of 3 hours, up to a maximum of five doses in total. If a lubricant is required with either of these preparations, a water-based lubricant jelly (such as KY Jelly®, Johnson & Johnson) should be used, not chlorhexidine cream (such as Hibitane Obstetric® cream, Centra-pharm), as this can inhibit absorption of the prostaglandin. The relative contraindications to prostaglandin treatment are:

- moderate to severe asthma
- allergy or previous hyperstimulation with prostaglandins
- previous uterine surgery.

All women with previous uterine surgery (such as caesarean section) must be discussed with senior medical staff. For such women, particularly at 22 weeks of gestation or above, the above treatment regimen may need to be altered.

It has been shown, using the above regimen of misoprostol (at gestations of 13–20 weeks) that abortion will be achieved in up to 97% of women. The prostaglandin induction-to-abortion time was 6 hours and 62% of women aborted following two doses of misoprostol. The women should be fasted after the administration of the first pessary and intravenous fluids commenced if abortion has not occurred by 8 hours after the first pessary. Most women find the procedure painful and distressing and require opiate analgesia. Normally this should be prescribed as diamorphine 5–10 mg intramuscularly, 3-hourly as required for pain. Non-steroidal anti-inflammatory drugs should be avoided.

At the time of discharge, the woman must be given anti-D if she is Rh-negative. The dosage varies according to gestation: 250 iu for gestations below 20 weeks and 500 iu for gestations at or above 20 weeks. A Kleihauer test should be performed to ensure that the dose given is adequate.

Bromocriptine should be administered from 20 weeks of gestation to suppress lactation, 2.5 mg on the first day, followed by 2.5 mg twice daily for 14 days. The general practitioner must be informed of the woman's discharge. Appropriate follow-up arrangements should be made with the GP, the patient's consultant or the prepregnancy clinic if required.

Late termination of pregnancy for fetal abnormality

Late diagnosis of fetal abnormality may occur as a result of:

- booking late in pregnancy
- an abnormality being missed earlier
- a disorder only diagnosable late in pregnancy; for example, achondroplasia, some forms of genetic microcephaly, severe growth restriction with organ failure or intracranial haemorrhage such as may occur with alloimmune thrombocytopenia or late viral infection with cytomegalovirus.

Such a diagnosis may lead to psychological harm or mental illness in the mother if she unwillingly continues with the pregnancy, delivers an unwanted child and then has the difficulty of rearing or sending for adoption a baby who is handicapped. The questions raised are whether these interests are grave enough to warrant late termination of pregnancy and whether unwillingness to rear a severely handicapped infant is a morally persuasive reason for termination. These issues and case examples are found in the RCOG publication on termination of pregnancy for fetal abnormality.[4] The recommendations of this and a further working party report on fetal awareness[5] state that if termination is to be carried out after 21^{+6} weeks, feticide should be carried out using a technique such as intracardiac injection of potassium chloride, which stops the fetal heart rapidly, with premedication being given to the mother, allowing time for it to build up in the fetus. The dose of potassium chloride chosen should ensure that fetal asystole has been achieved. This should be confirmed by observing the fetal heart for a period of up to 5 minutes. It is also recommended that asystole is confirmed by a further ultrasound examination 30–60 minutes after the procedure and certainly before the woman leaves the hospital. The RCOG report concluded that 'the use of analgesia provided no clear benefit to the fetus' and 'fetal analgesia should not be employed where the only consideration is concern about fetal awareness or pain'.[4] There is no clear benefit in considering the need for fetal analgesia prior to termination of pregnancy, even after 24 weeks, in cases of fetal abnormality.[4]

Both documents make a clear statement that it is particularly important for referring clinicians to have early discussions with a specialist in fetal medicine to confirm the diagnosis and to arrange appropriate management.[4,5] Late feticides should be carried out by trained fetal medicine specialists in recognised fetal medicine centres. Such facilities should have agreed multidisciplinary management plans in place before late termination is arranged. These plans should take in to account issues such as conscientious objection. The multidisciplinary team should include, where appropriate, obstetricians, neonatologists, geneticists and midwives. If the fetus has a lethal abnormality and the woman decides not to undergo feticide, there must be a clear management plan in place for the fetus after birth. These plans should take into account the recommendations of the British Association of Perinatal Medicine surrounding the management of fetuses and newborns at the threshold of viability.[6]

Multifetal pregnancy reduction

Perinatal outcome is significantly poorer in high-order multiple pregnancies, mainly because of preterm delivery and low birth weight. As a consequence of these complications, the rates of cerebral palsy are estimated to be four times that of singletons.[7] It is also important to be aware of the increased maternal risk with multiple pregnancies, many of which also occur in women of advanced maternal age, a further substantial maternal and fetal risk factor.[8]

Multifetal pregnancy reduction was developed about 20 years ago in an attempt to diminish these adverse sequelae.[9] It is normally carried out between 11and 14 weeks of gestation. Collaborative data from centres with the most experience have shown that multifetal pregnancy reduction can be performed with essentially 100% technical success rate, leading to improved survival and decreased morbidity of fetuses after reduction than there would have been in the high-order multiple births without reduction. Two main techniques have resulted:

- transabdominal needle insertion for injection of intrathoracic potassium chloride
- transvaginal or transcervical aspiration or mechanical disruption of the embryo.

The transvaginal route was associated with a higher loss rate (12% compared with 5.4% for the transabdominal route). The transabdominal technique requires a thorough ultrasound examination to document proper fetal number and to look for any fetal abnormalities. Measurement of nuchal translucency in each fetus should also be undertaken, with those fetuses having an increased measurement selected for fetal reduction in preference to those with a normal nuchal translucency measurement.[10] Fetuses demonstrating abnormalities should be selected for reduction but, in practice, it is those fetuses closest to the fundus of the uterus that are easier to reduce. The selection of the fetus furthest away from the cervix also reduces the risk of ascending infection in retained dead tissue. It is also important to look for the appearance of a presumed monozygotic twin pair and these two would be selected for reduction in preference to singletons.

One of the main controversial areas with multifetal pregnancy reduction concerns the data available on the reduction of triplet pregnancies. As no randomised studies have been performed in this area, the only data available are those of a meta-analysis of 14 studies of reduced triplets and 17 of unreduced triplets. This has suggested that there was a non-significant reduction in pregnancy loss below 24 weeks with reduced triplets compared with unreduced triplets (5.7% compared with 7.5%). The meta-analysis also showed a lower preterm delivery rate below 28 and 32 weeks in the reduced triplets. This led to a lower perinatal mortality rate in the reduced triplets (43/1000 compared with 110/1000 live births).[11] These data suggest that reduction of triplets to twins reduces the early preterm delivery rate towards that of unreduced twins. A woman with a triplet pregnancy thus should be counselled and offered multifetal pregnancy reduction. This difficult decision can be made even more complex by the offering of reduction to a singleton pregnancy. This further reduction can lower the risk of preterm delivery even further but it does come at the expense of an increased miscarriage rate. There is evidence that couples are more prepared now to reduce triplets to singleton pregnancies.[12]

TECHNICAL ASPECTS

The abdomen is washed and draped in the usual manner. Using ultrasound, with or without a biopsy attachment, a spot on the abdomen directly above the sac to be entered is chosen and a 22-gauge needle is inserted through the abdominal wall in a directly vertical approach. Once the needle is in the appropriate sac, it is manoeuvred directly over the thorax of the fetus. This insertion must be done briskly since, if pushed slowly, the embryo will merely be pushed out of the way. Once the operator is satisfied that the needle is inside the thorax, the stilette is removed and the syringe with potassium chloride is attached to the end of the needle. The potassium is injected slowly since, if it is inserted too rapidly, this can push the fetus off the tip of the needle. Generally, 0.5–1.0 ml is

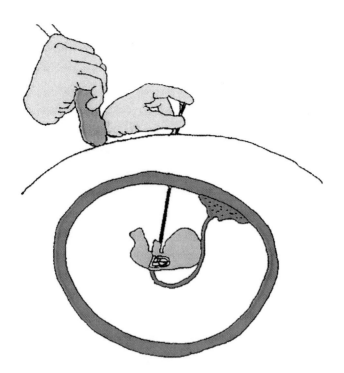

Figure 7.1 Technique used in multifetal pregnancy reduction

required to ensure cardiac asystole. The needle should be kept in place to make sure there is no reinitiation of cardiac activity. A new needle is used and the next fetus is then selected in an identical fashion (Figure 7.1).

SELECTIVE TERMINATION

The option of selective termination is available to a mother who has been diagnosed as having one twin with a serious fetal abnormality. Such cases require careful evaluation of the fetal anatomy, followed by a detailed counselling session explaining the underlying diagnosis and the options available. Establishing the diagnosis, providing counselling and performing the techniques should be undertaken in an experienced fetal medicine centre. The first major concern is to ensure that the correct fetus is selected. Although high-resolution ultrasound has made it rare that an abnormal fetus, even one with a chromosomal abnormality, has no detectable morphologic anomalies, occasionally this is still the case. Under these circumstances, it is critical to ensure that the documentation from the laboratory and from the first ultrasound scan under which the amniocentesis or chorionic villus sampling was performed is consistent with what is observed. Also, placental position must be observed and a demarcation made between the placentas, to reduce the likelihood of either of the injected potassium chloride or coagulation products affecting the other twin.

A 20-gauge spinal needle is inserted transabdominally directly over the fetal thorax under sterile conditions. The needle should be placed directly into the fetal cardiac chamber and the return of blood seen. Once the needle has been correctly positioned, approximately 2 ml of potassium chloride is injected over 20 seconds. This will usually produce cardiac asystole. However, depending on the gestational age, another 1–7 ml may sometimes be necessary. The needle should not be removed until cardiac asystole is confirmed.

The safety of selective termination depends on lack of vascular communication between the fetuses. Based on reports from the international registry, the rate of preterm delivery following intracardiac potassium chloride is relatively low: 12% at gestations less than 33 weeks and 6% at less than 28 weeks of gestation.[13] However, the technique described above is not appropriate where there is monochorionic placentation. In such circumstances, a number of vaso-occlusive techniques, including bipolar cord occlusion or radiofrequency ablation, have been used.[14] Such cases also require referral to a tertiary fetal medicine centre.

Conclusion

Termination of pregnancy for fetal abnormality is a sensitive and emotive subject that leads to a great deal of moral and ethical debate.[15] Health professionals involved in this area have a pivotal role. They should give sympathetic, supportive and accurate non-directive counselling concerning the specific abnormality that has been identified. In addition they should provide a supportive role for the couple once their decision has been made. A further role is to organise up-to-date protocols that deliver an efficient and safe method of terminating the pregnancy. Follow up is essential in order that a bereavement counselling appointment can be made. At this meeting a sensitive debriefing of the fetal diagnosis and recurrence risks should be discussed, together with a clear plan of management for any future pregnancy.

References

1. Fisher J, Statham H. Parental reaction to prenatal diagnosis and subsequent bereavement. In: *Fetal Medicine: Basic Science and Clinical Practice*. Rodeck CH, Whittle MJ, editors. London: Churchill Livingstone; 2008. p. 234–42.

2. Royal College of Obstetricians and Gynaecologists. *The Care of Women Requesting Induced Abortion*. Evidence-based Guideline No. 7. London: RCOG Press; 2004 [www.rcog.org.uk/womens-health/clinical-guidance/care-women-requesting-induced-abortion].

3. Kalish RB, Chasen ST, Rosenzweig LB, Rashbaum WK, Chervenak FA. Impact of mid-trimester dilation and evacuation on subsequent pregnancy outcome. *Am J Obstet Gynecol* 2002;187:882–5.

4. Royal College of Obstetricians and Gynaecologists. *Termination of Pregnancy for Fetal Abnormality in England, Scotland and Wales: Report of a Working Party*. London: RCOG; 2010 [www.rcog.org.uk/termination-pregnancy-fetal-abnormality-england-scotland-and-wales].

5. Royal College of Obstetricians and Gynaecologists. *Fetal Awareness: Review of Research and Recommendations for Practice. Report of a Working Party*. London: RCOG; 2010 [www.rcog.org.uk/fetal-awareness-review-research-and-recommendation-practice].

6. British Association of Perinatal Medicine; Gee H, Dunn PM. *Fetuses and Newborn Infants at the Threshold of Viability: A Framework for Practice*. BAPM Memorandum. London: BAPM; November 1999 [www.bapm.org/documents/publications/threshold.pdf].

7. Topp M, Huusom LD, Langhoff- Roos J, Delhumeau C, Hutton JL, Dolk H; SCPE Collaborative Group. Multiple birth and cerebral palsy in Europe: a multicentre study. *Acta Obstet Gynecol Scand* 2004;83:548–53.

8. Luke B, Brown MB. Contemporary risks of maternal morbidity and adverse outcomes with increasing maternal age and plurality. *Fertil Steril* 2007;88:283–93.

9. Berkowitz RL, Lynch L, Chitkara U, Wilkins IA, Mehalek KE, Alvarez E. Selective reduction of multifetal pregnancies in the first trimester. *N Engl J Med* 1988;318:1043–47.

10. Evans MI, Ciorica D, Britt DW, Fletcher JC. Update on selective reduction. *Prenat Diagn* 2005;25:807–13.

11. Wimalasundera R. Selective reduction and termination of multiple pregnancies. In: *Multiple Pregnancy*. Kilby MBP, Critchley H, Field D, editors. London: RCOG Press; 2006. p. 89–108.

12. Stone J, Belogolovkin V, Matho A, Berkowitz RL, Moshier E, Eddleman K. Evolving trends in 2000 cases of multifetal pregnancy reduction: a single center experience. *Am J Obstet Gynecol* 2007;197:394;e1–4.

13. Evans MI, Goldberg JD, Horenstein J, Wapner RJ, Ayoub MA, Stone J, *et al.* Selective termination for structural, chromosomal, and Mendelian anomalies: international experience. *Am J Obstet Gynecol* 1999;181:893–7.

14. Klaritsch P, Albert K, Van Mieghem T, Gucciardo L, Done' E, Bynens B, *et al.* Instrumental requirements for minimally invasive fetal surgery. *BJOG* 2009;116:188–97.

15. Wicks E, Wyldes M, Kilby M. Late termination of pregnancy for fetal abnormality: medical and legal perspectives. *Med Law Rev* 2004;12:285–305

8 Fetal growth restriction

Introduction

Five to ten percent of pregnancies result in the delivery of a small neonate. The majority are simply statistically small for their gestational age; they have grown at a constant velocity and are otherwise healthy. A minority are born small because growth during the pregnancy has been restricted. Growth restriction may be caused by one of many pathological processes (Table 8.1) but not infrequently while there is neonatal evidence of intrauterine starvation (dry wrinkled skin, loss of adipose tissue and muscle wasting) no specific aetiology can be identified to account for the growth restriction. These cases of 'unexplained' fetal growth restriction are the clinical manifestation of a pathological process that occurs in the placenta during the first half of pregnancy, which results in inadequate fetal nutrition. This chapter reviews normal and abnormal placental development, assessment of the growth-restricted fetus and outlines investigations and treatment strategies that may be used in subsequent pregnancies.

Table 8.1   Pathological causes of fetal growth restriction

Causes of SGA pregnancies	Pathology
Chromosome anomalies	Triploidy Trisomy 21, 18, 13
Congenital infection	First-trimester exposure to rubella Cytomegalovirus Toxoplasmosis
Structural abnormalities	Skeletal dysplasias Dwarfism Gastroschisis
Teratogens	First-trimester exposure to warfarin Fetal alcohol syndrome

SGA = small for gestational age

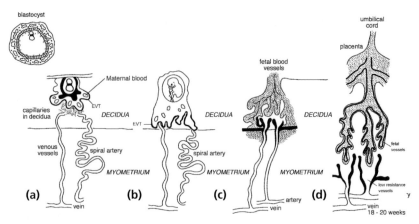

Figure 8.1 Placental development: (a) and (b) the blastocyst implants, extravillous trophoblast (EVT) invades the maternal decidua; (c) & (d) with further invasion, the it converts the spiral arteries into flaccid vessels giving a rich blood supply to the villi. A rich network of fetal vessels within each villous branch ensures rapid transfer of nutrients between mother and fetus

Normal uteroplacental development

The fertilised ovum undergoes multiple cell divisions as it migrates to the uterine cavity and forms the blastocyst. The blastocyst adheres to the endometrium and, by a process of controlled breakdown of the extracellular matrix involving metalloproteinases and cell adhesion molecules, implants the early pregnancy firmly within the endometrial stroma.

Implantation is complete by 10–12 days post-fertilisation. The conceptus must then establish a long-term link with the maternal circulation to secure an adequate nutritional supply and facilitate further growth of the pregnancy. This process of placentation (the formation of the placenta) will provide the interface between mother and baby until the time of delivery (Figure 8.1).

DEVELOPMENT OF UTEROPLACENTAL BLOOD SUPPLY

During the first trimester, fingerlike projections of trophoblast cells, known as extravillous trophoblasts, invade the maternal uterine stroma, extending as far as the decidual–myometrial junction. As the trophoblast invasion extends, small maternal vessels or capillaries within the decidua are engulfed. These tiny lakes of maternal blood within the developing trophoblast provide initial nutrition to the conceptus (Figure 8.1a,b). In the absence of a formal blood supply, these primitive or early placental villi develop within a relatively avascular environment at low oxygen tensions.

As the depth of invasion increases, the extravillous trophoblasts encounter larger-diameter arterioles. These vessels are initially surrounded then occluded with plugs of extravillous trophoblast cells. Sometime around the end of the first trimester (week 10–12) the extravillous trophoblast plugs loosen and maternal blood begins to flow freely into the intervillous space, draining back to the maternal circulation via spiral venules (Figure 8.1c). Direct transfer of oxygen and nutrients occurs from the maternal blood across the trophoblast interface to the fetal circulation. With the acquisition of a formal maternal vascular supply to the developing placenta, oxygen tension around the villi rises dramatically. This timely process is essential for successful pregnancy outcome.

At around 16–18 weeks of gestation, the extravillous trophoblast invades deeper into the myometrium, surrounding larger spiral arteries in the process. The extravillous trophoblast induces fibrinoid change within the muscular walls of the spiral arteries. With the destruction of the elastic media and muscle, the spiral arteries are incapable of vasoactive responsiveness. The muscularised resistance vessels soon become flaccid tubes that easily accommodate the increased blood flow to the placental bed (Figure 8.1d). Modification of the spiral arteries is usually complete by week 24, at the end of the second trimester. Invasion of the developing trophoblast into the maternal decidua and myometrium is regulated by a variety of growth factors and adhesion molecules.

DEVELOPMENT OF THE PLACENTAL VILLOUS STRUCTURE

Placental villous and vascular development is intimately linked and occurs concurrently. Following implantation, the fetoplacental circulation develops from haemangioblastic stem cells. These cells initially merge together to form primitive capillary vessels within the developing trophoblast villi. Under the influence of angiogenic and other growth factors, such as vascular endothelial growth factor (VEGF) and placental growth factor (PlGF), the placental vessels enlarge and divide multiple times, forming an elaborate network of vessels within the villi.

As invasion into the maternal myometrium progresses, the trophoblast cells are likewise replicating to form multiple small villous branches (tertiary villi) that grow out from the main stem villi. This tree-like structure of trophoblast villi increases the surface area for fetomaternal exchange dramatically. This, in conjunction with the extensive network of capillary vessels within each villous branch, allows rapid transfer of nutrients and waste products between mother and fetus (Figure 8.1d).

Uteroplacental development in fetal growth restriction

Both uteroplacental blood flow and the mean placental weight are reduced in pregnancies complicated by severe growth restriction. This is because of a combination of factors, namely primary maldevelopment of the placenta and impaired adaptation of the maternal circulation.

UTEROPLACENTAL BLOOD FLOW

Inadequate invasion of the maternal myometrium by extravillous trophoblast cells allows maternal spiral arteries to retain a muscular, vasoactive vessel wall. As a result, blood flow to the placental bed is restricted and, as a consequence, nutritional supplies to the fetoplacental unit are limited. While this constraint may be tolerated by the early conceptus and pregnancy progress may be apparently normally, with advancing gestation the deficit becomes pronounced and fetal growth is impaired to varying degrees. Hysterectomy specimens and placental-bed biopsies from pregnancies affected by severe growth restriction clearly demonstrate failure of spiral artery remodelling. In severe cases of fetal growth restriction, uteroplacental blood flow may be reduced by as much as 50%.

PLACENTAL VILLOUS DEVELOPMENT

Development of the placental villous tree is also abnormal in pregnancies with severe fetal growth restriction. For reasons that remain unclear, the complex network of tertiary villi that should form during the second and third trimesters and offer a large and effective area for gas and nutrient exchange, fails to develop adequately. In addition, the rich vascular capillary network that usually occupies the tertiary villi is virtually absent. In combination, these factors result in a small, poorly perfused placental unit that has a significantly diminished surface area for nutrient and gas exchange. These constraints place the fetus in 'starvation' mode and, as a consequence, fetal growth patterns are modified. There is a growing body of evidence to suggest that pregnancies complicated by severe fetal growth restriction have reduced levels of the angiogenic factors VEGF and PlGF. This may explain the restricted vascular network within the placental villi. Factors associated with impaired trophoblast invasion, namely soluble fms-like tyrosine kinase, are also increased, possibly restricting villous development and, as a consequence, reducing the degree of uterine invasion.

Antenatal features of growth-restricted pregnancies

In the absence of a previous history or coexistent maternal disease, most pregnancies with fetal growth restriction present with clinical evidence of a small-for-dates uterus and/or reduced fetal movements in the second half of pregnancy. Ultrasound-derived estimates of fetal size using head circumference, abdominal circumference and femur length can confirm an estimated fetal weight. The majority of centres restrict the use of small-for-dates uterus to those pregnancies with an estimated abdominal circumference or estimated fetal weight less than the fifth centile. This group will also include many babies that are constitutionally small but not compromised. Distinguishing the fetus that is small but healthy from one that is starved *in utero* and at high risk is a challenge. Additional assessments, such as amniotic fluid volume, Doppler studies and cardiotocography, must then be used to assess the fetal condition and to plan the timing of delivery (Figure 8.2).

Assessment of the small fetus

AMNIOTIC FLUID VOLUME

During the second half of pregnancy, fetal urine is the main source of amniotic fluid. Amniotic fluid is swallowed by the fetus, absorbed from the fetal gut into the bloodstream then circulated through the renal glomeruli to produce more fetal urine. In the absence of premature

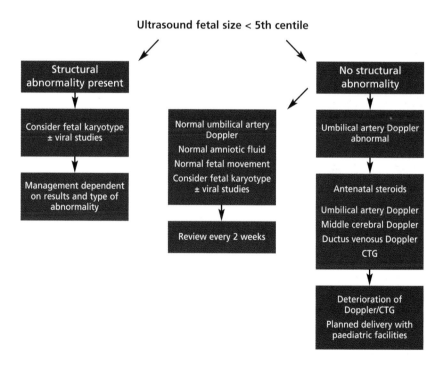

Figure 8.2 The role of ultrasound in the management of a fetus found to be clinically small for gestational age; CTG = cardiotography

rupture of the membranes or structural abnormalities in the fetal kidneys, reduced levels of amniotic fluid are thought to reflect impaired renal perfusion. Renal blood flow is reduced if the fetus is hypoxic or hypovolaemic, as blood flow is prioritised to vital organs such as the heart and the brain at the expense of non-essential organs such as the kidneys. Reduced amniotic fluid volumes are therefore an indirect measure of placental function and fetal hypoxia, particularly in the preterm fetus. An amniotic fluid index of less than 5 cm is thought to be significant.

DOPPLER WAVEFORMS

Doppler ultrasound permits non-invasive *in vivo* evaluation of fetal blood flow patterns by using the Doppler principle. This states that a sound wave reflected from a moving target, such as blood cells, will return at a different frequency from the incident wave emitted. The change in sound wave frequency, which is proportional to the velocity of the moving object, is known as the frequency shift or Doppler shift.[1]

In arterial vessels, blood flow is more rapid during systole than in diastole while in veins, blood flow is generally constant throughout the cardiac cycle. There are also differences within vessels. Blood flow in the centre of a vessel is more rapid than blood flow near the vessel wall. At any one point in a vessel, there is a spectrum of frequency shifts, each reflecting different blood flow velocity. All these measurements are recorded, averaged by computer and plotted against time to produce a smooth waveform known as the flow velocity waveform (FVW).

A qualitative assessment of blood flow within the fetoplacental circulation may be derived from the diastolic component of the FVW. This portion of the FVW reflects downstream impedance within the vessel being examined and is independent of any other variable such as fetal size or blood volume. Several indices have been used to describe the FVW (Box 8.1).

Standard tables of the normal ranges for each ratio at each gestational age are available for most of the major fetal vessels. All three indices are highly correlated.

BOX 8.1 INDICES DESCRIBING THE FLOW VELOCITY WAVEFORM

A/B or S/D ratio	the ratio of peak systolic (S) to maximal diastolic (D) flow velocity
Resistance index (RI)	S – D/S
Pulsatility index (PI)	S – D/mean velocity

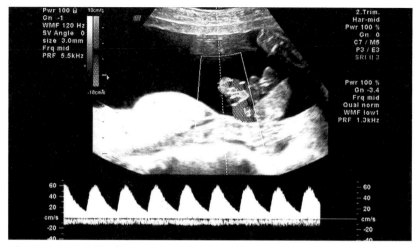

Figure 8.3 Umbilical artery Doppler waveform in normal pregnancy, showing a large diastolic component

Umbilical artery Doppler waveforms

Placental vascular impedance falls with advancing gestation in normal pregnancy. This permits the enlarging fetal blood volume to circulate freely through the placenta and ensures that adequate nutritional substrates are extracted from the maternal circulation to supply the growing fetus. The large diastolic component seen in the umbilical FVW reflects this low impedance to blood flow (Figure 8.3).

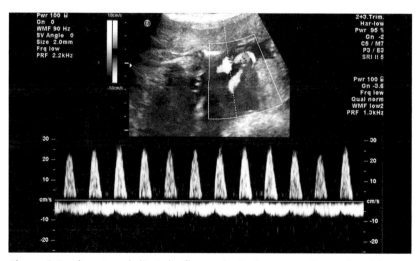

Figure 8.4 Absent end-diastolic flow velocity in a growth-restricted fetus

In pregnancies complicated by severe fetal growth restriction, the diastolic component of the FVW is firstly reduced (increasing pulsatility index, PI) then absent and finally reversed (Figure 8.4). These changes reflect increasing placental vascular impedance and reduced placental perfusion. Perinatal morbidity and mortality are directly correlated with the progressive changes of reduced/absent/reversed diastolic flow velocity in the umbilical artery waveform. Increasing umbilical artery PI is usually the first indication that a small fetus is compensating for inadequate nutrition and oxygen.

Middle cerebral artery Doppler waveforms

During normal pregnancy, cerebral impedance decreases with advancing gestation, facilitating an increase in cerebral blood flow to the growing fetus. Doppler studies of the fetal middle cerebral artery (MCA) reflect this change, such that the end-diastolic flow velocity increases and PI measurements fall.

In pregnancies affected by severe fetal growth restriction, the fetus must maintain cerebral blood flow, even at the expense of other organs: the 'brain-sparing' effect. This can only be done by reducing cerebral vascular impedance. The Doppler waveform will show increased diastolic flow, reflected by low PI measurements. As hypoxia progresses however, maximal cerebral vasodilatation is reached and no further compensation possible. Beyond this nadir, further hypoxia results only in severe cerebral vasoconstriction, probably from cerebral oedema. This may be seen as an apparent return to 'normal' PI recordings but is in fact a sinister sign. For this reason, an individual PI reading may be difficult to interpret: is it truly normal or an ominous sign? The MCA peak systolic velocity (PSV) may prove to be a more useful marker. Some groups have recently found this to rise progressively and consistently with deterioration of the fetal condition (Figure 8.5). Tables of the normal values for gestational age are available.[2]

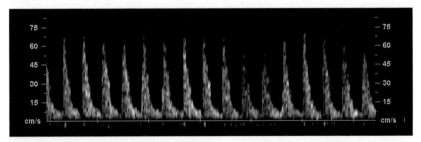

Figure 8.5 Middle cerebral artery peak systolic velocity above 50 cm/second in a growth-restricted fetus at 26 weeks of gestation

Ductus venosus waveform

The ductus venosus arises from the umbilical vein and enters the inferior vena cava just below the diaphragm. Approximately 40% of blood in the umbilical vein is directed via the ductus venosus through the inferior vena cava and into the heart. Within the inferior vena cava, blood from the ductus venosus is preferentially directed through the foramen ovale into the left atrium and from there to the fetal heart, brain and other organs. There are three distinct portions to the flow velocity waveform in the normally grown fetus (Figure 8.6) reflecting cardiac systole, diastole and atrial contraction. In the normally grown fetus, there is forward flow velocity during the entire cardiac cycle.

In unfavourable fetal conditions, such as reduced umbilical venous pressure, increased fetal haematocrit and fetal hypoxia, umbilical venous blood flow is preferentially directed through the ductus venosus at the expense of other organs such as the liver and lower abdominal structures. These circulatory changes are reflected in the altered flow velocity waveforms that ensue. The flow waveforms show a highly pulsatile pattern with increased peak systolic flow and retrograde flow during atrial contraction. Abnormalities in the ductus venosus waveform are strongly correlated with fetal acidaemia.[3,4]

Umbilical vein waveform

Flow velocity in the umbilical vein should be evaluated just before it enters the fetal abdomen. In normal pregnancy, there is continuous forward flow in the umbilical vein although, during periods of fetal breathing, this may

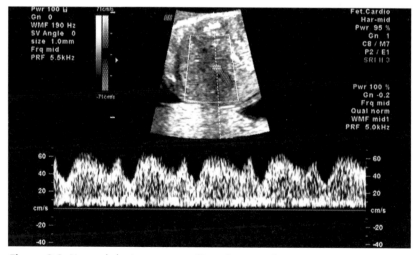

Figure 8.6 Normal ductus venosus Doppler waveform

undulate. In the compromised fetus, as peripheral vasoconstriction intensifies and venous pressures increase, there is a reduction of velocity at end-diastole in the umbilical vein resulting in a pulsatile pattern. These changes are strongly associated with fetal acidaemia.

Cardiotocography

Antenatal recordings of fetal heart rate patterns are a subjective assessment of fetal wellbeing. A reactive cardiotocogram (CTG) is strongly associated with a good perinatal outcome but numerous studies have demonstrated that almost 50% of the recordings deemed to be non-reassuring are still associated with good outcome and just as many of those thought to be reassuring had a poor outcome. In the presence of severe fetal growth restriction, with increasing fetal hypoxia and academia, the fetal heart pattern changes. Fetal activity is reduced and accelerations disappear. As hypoxia worsens, baseline variability diminishes and decelerations appear. Poor short-term variability is highly correlated with fetal academia.

Optimal time to deliver the growth-restricted fetus

To identify the optimal time for delivery, several studies have attempted to establish the sequence of change that occurs as the growth-restricted fetus progressively compensates. Disappointingly, not all cases of growth restriction follow the same pattern of deterioration and there is therefore no single test that best determines the optimal time to deliver a growth restricted fetus. Confounding variables, such as maternal hypertension, pre-eclampsia and diabetes, can all affect the onset and rate of fetal compromise. However, studies have consistently shown that perinatal survival is highly correlated with gestational age at delivery. For this reason, in growth-restricted pregnancies of less than 30 weeks of gestation, delaying delivery, ideally until at least 28 weeks of gestation, providing Doppler and CTG assessments of the fetus are stable, it highly advantageous.

In general, Doppler changes in the fetal circulation occur in the sequence shown in Figure 8.7. Changes in amniotic fluid volumes and CTG patterns are less predictable and occur at varying times within this sequence of events.

In the small fetus with reduced end-diastolic flow velocity but otherwise normal monitoring, weekly review should be sufficient. Once end-diastolic flow is absent, increased fetal surveillance should be initiated. The frequency of review will vary between institutions but should be at least three times a week. Timing of delivery should be individualised, based on the clinical situation and signs of worsening compromise, as

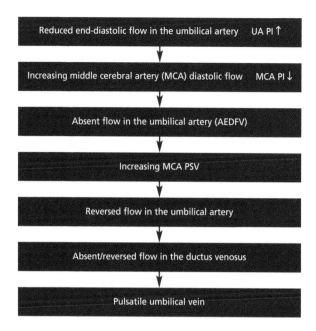

Figure 8.7 Doppler changes in fetal circulation

evidenced by Doppler/CTG studies. There is a pressing need for a well controlled randomised study to assess the timing of delivery in relation to these Doppler changes.

In pregnancies over 34 weeks of gestation, the finding of abnormal umbilical artery Doppler would usually prompt delivery, even if other Doppler studies are normal,[5] as there is little fetal benefit to be gained in delaying delivery.

Neonatal effects of fetal growth restriction

Growth restriction *in utero* predisposes the neonate to complications of low birth weight and, if preterm delivery is required, the added complications of prematurity.

THERMOREGULATION

The growth-restricted infant has a low ponderal index. As body length is usually preserved, there is a large surface area present, through which heat loss can occur. The lack of subcutaneous adipose tissue, high basal metabolic rates and thin permeable skin that characterise such infants, accelerate the rate at which heat loss occurs. Hypothermia increases neonatal caloric expenditure and the risks of metabolic acidosis. It is therefore vital that these babies are dried and maintained in a warm environment following delivery.

HYPOGLYCAEMIA

The transition from fetal to neonatal life is associated with risks of hypoglycaemia. The deposits of glycogen and lipids laid down in fetal life usually ensure that a steady supply of substrates is available and fasting sugar levels are maintained. Growth-restricted neonates, however, have little adipose tissue and so have depleted stores of lipids and glycogen. In addition, increased insulin levels and impaired gluconeogenesis, metabolic adaptations to the poor fetal environment, restrict the growth-restricted neonate's ability to cope further. Episodes of hypoglycaemia, if allowed to occur, are strongly associated with adverse neurological outcome. Blood glucose levels must therefore be monitored regularly and early/frequent feeding encouraged.

POLYCYTHAEMIA

In the presence of chronic hypoxia *in utero*, the fetus must maximise oxygen availability. One mechanism by which this is achieved is an increase in red cell mass. *In utero*, erythropoietin levels and red cell production are directly correlated to the degree of antenatal fetal compromise. As a consequence, fetal haematocrit and blood viscosity at birth are increased in severely growth-restricted fetuses.[4] Most neonates will remain asymptomatic but increased blood viscosity may well compromise blood flow within the microvessels of the gut and brain, leading to increased risks of necrotising enterocolitis and cerebral events.

COMPLICATIONS OF PREMATURITY

Severely growth-restricted neonates are frequently delivered prematurely. When compared with appropriate for gestational age neonates, growth-restricted neonates have an increased incidence of chronic respiratory problems, necrotising enterocolitis and intraventricular haemorrhage. Increased fetal blood viscosity, redirection of blood flow from the gut to vital organs like the heart, consequent reperfusion injury of these organs following delivery and increased oxygen free radicals may all contribute to this problem.

Prediction of fetal growth restriction

Vigorous attempts have been made to identify those women at risk of placental growth problems later in pregnancy. Pulsed Doppler analysis of the uterine arteries is an indirect assessment of impedance within the

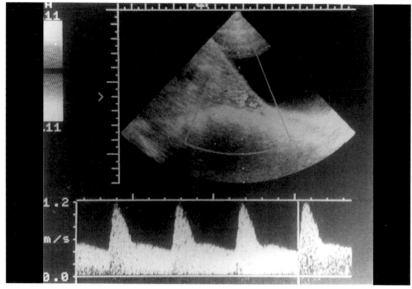

(a)

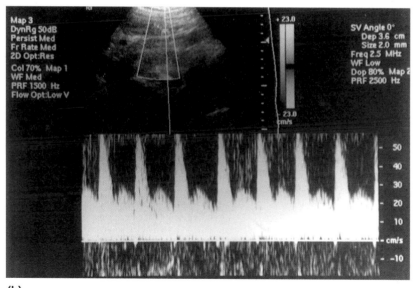

(b)

Figure 8.8 Uterine artery Doppler waveform: (a) normal waveform with a smooth diastolic component; (b) waveform at 24 weeks in a woman with a previous pregnancy affected by fetal growth restriction and pre-eclampsia; the diastolic notch is still present

uteroplacental circulation. In normal pregnancy, uteroplacental impedance falls in the second trimester, with the conversion of muscularised spiral arterioles into flaccid vessels. The resulting uterine artery waveform shows a large smooth diastolic component (Figure 8.8a). Where uteroplacental impedance remains elevated, owing to failure of spiral artery remodelling, the resistance index increases and a 'notch' appears during the diastolic component of the waveform (Figure 8.8b).

Uterine artery Doppler studies have been performed at 20–24 weeks of gestation, in both high- and low-risk populations, in an attempt to predict those at risk of fetal growth restriction.[7-9] Normal uterine artery Doppler studies in the second trimester are very reassuring and usually result in a good pregnancy outcome. However, the positive predictive value of an abnormal uterine artery Doppler examination, even in high-risk populations, in the second trimester remains poor, with figures consistently less than 30%.

Given the limited value of Doppler studies, other potential tests have been explored. Both in animal and human studies, low levels of pregnancy-associated plasma protein A in the first trimester are associated with risks of fetal growth restriction and stillbirth. Elevated serum alphafetoprotein levels in the second trimester are also associated with complications of fetal growth. These two variables appear to be independent markers. With the introduction of two-staged screening programmes, it is possible that, in the future, these markers may be used either independently or in conjunction with Doppler studies to highlight those women at most risk of restricted fetal growth.

Potential therapies for fetal growth restriction

Poor fetal growth *in utero* is thought to be caused by a lack of oxygen and substrates *in utero*, secondary to poor uteroplacental blood flow and abnormal placental development. Each of these areas has been explored in an attempt to find potential means of preventing and/or treating idiopathic growth restriction.

OXYGEN THERAPY

Umbilical venous oxygen levels are significantly lower in growth-restricted fetuses. A few small studies have given mothers with growth-restricted pregnancies supplemental oxygen in an attempt to improve the fetal oxygen levels. While initial results were encouraging, there are concerns about the safety of this treatment. Prolonged oxygen exposure restricts maternal movement and the long-term effects on maternal lung function are unclear. In addition, some animal work has suggested that the growth-restricted fetus cannot use additional oxygen, the lower fetal levels reflecting the limited capability of the placenta to transfer oxygen, rather than the maternal supply. If supplemental maternal oxygen is then discontinued for any reason, there is a rebound period of worsening fetal oxygenation and serious risk to the fetus.

NUTRITIONAL THERAPY

To improve the availability of substrates to the growth-restricted fetus, various regimens using glucose, protein, vitamins and minerals, either orally or by infusion, have been investigated. To date, none has proved effective in improving fetal growth and some, such as intravenous maternal glucose, have proved hazardous to the fetus, resulting in acidosis.

IMPROVING UTEROPLACENTAL BLOOD FLOW

Uteroplacental blood flow is thought to improve with maternal rest. At present, there is no conclusive evidence of improved fetal growth with maternal rest. Given the maternal risks of prolonged bed rest, such as deep venous thrombosis, prolonged maternal rest is not recommended for mothers with growth-restricted pregnancies.

Aspirin 60–150 mg daily is known to inhibit platelet cyclooxygenase and the production of thromboxane, a potent vasoconstrictor. Given the persistence of vasoactive spiral arteries in pregnancies complicated by fetal growth restriction, aspirin has been used with a view to reduce the degree of vasospasm present in the spiral arteries and to reduce platelet aggregation within the uterine circulation, thus improving blood flow to the placental bed.

The introduction of low-dose aspirin therapy to pregnancies already affected by fetal growth restriction or to those with significant risk factors such as abnormal uterine artery Doppler at 24 weeks of gestation, does not appear to improve fetal growth or fetal outcome. The changes in placental and uterine blood flow already appear to be well established by 24 weeks of gestation and do not appear to be reversible. Aspirin, used from the first trimester onwards, may have a role in preventing fetal growth restriction in later pregnancies, although the exact mechanism for this remains unclear.

Long-term sequelae of restricted fetal growth in utero

Multiple studies in a wide range of groups have clearly demonstrated that poor fetal growth and patterns of growth in the first few years of life have consequences for later adult health. The incidence of hypertension in adult life rises as birth weight falls and death from cardiovascular disease is strongly correlated with a low ponderal index at birth. Serum cholesterol and low-density lipoprotein concentrations, both additional cardiovascular risk factors, are elevated in adults who were low-birthweight babies. At least two hypotheses have been proposed to explain these findings. Firstly, an adverse fetal environment may influence the development of key organs and structures, with subsequent long term effects. Babies of low birth weight tend to have a reduced number of renal nephrons, which could affect renal function and blood pressure control in later life. Secondly, an adverse fetal environment may 'set' hormone or messenger pathways. If there is a depleted supply of substrates, relative insulin resistance *in utero* will maintain circulating glucose levels but will reduce muscle growth. *In utero*, this will be a useful means of protecting organs such as the brain but, if it is maintained into newborn and childhood life, patterns of carbohydrate handling will be adversely 'set'. There is also evidence to suggest that people who were small at birth have higher cortisol levels and are therefore less able to deal with adverse environmental influences during life. The exact interactions between fetal, neonatal, childhood and adult disease patterns are still being evaluated and increasingly appear to be interlinked. Patterns of growth *in utero* play a key role in the outcome of subsequent adult health.

Summary

Idiopathic fetal growth restriction is the clinical manifestation of abnormal placental development in the first half of pregnancy. The diagnosis of a pregnancy with fetal growth restriction has significant implications for pregnancy and the long-term health of any surviving neonate.

Increasing fetal compromise can be assessed using an integrated assessment of several Doppler parameters but predicting the optimal time for delivery, when the fetal risks exceed that of a small, preterm neonate remains a challenge for all obstetricians.

References

1. Trudinger BJ, Giles WB, Cook CM, Bombardien J, Collins L. Fetal umbilical artery flow velocity waveforms and placental resistance: clinical significance. *Br J Obstet Gynaecol* 1985;92:23–30.

2. Mari G, Hanif F, Kruger M, Cosmi E, Santolaya-Forgas J, Treadwell MC. Middle cerebral artery peak systolic velocity: a new Doppler parameter in the assessment of growth-restricted fetuses. *Ultrasound Obstet Gynecol* 2007;29:310–16.

3. Baschat AA, Cosmi E, Bilardo CM, Wolf H, Berg C, Rigano S, *et al.* Predictors of neonatal outcome in early onset placental dysfunction. *Obstet Gynaecol* 2007;109:253–261.

4. Mari G, Hanif F, Treadwell MC, Kruger M. Gestational age at delivery and Doppler waveforms in very preterm intrauterine growth restricted fetuses as predictors of perinatal mortality. *J Ultrasound Med* 2007;26:555–559.

5. Royal College of Obstetricians and Gynaecologists. *The Investigation and Management of the Small-for-gestational-age Fetus*. Green-top Guideline No. 31. London: RCOG; 2002 [www.rcog.org.uk/womens-health/investigation-and-management-small-gestational-age-fetus-green-top-31].

6. Soothill P, Nicolaides KH, Campbell S. Prenatal asphyxia, hyperlacticemia, hypoglycemia and erythroblastosis in growth retarded fetuses. *BMJ* 1987;294:1051–3.

7. Bewley S, Cooper D, Campbell S. Doppler investigation of uteroplacental blood flow resistance in the second trimester: a screening study for pre-eclampsia and intrauterine growth retardation. *Br J Obstet Gynaecol* 1991;98:871–9.

8. Bower S, Schuchter K, Campbell S. Doppler ultrasound screening as part of routine antenatal scanning: prediction of pre-eclampsia and intrauterine growth retardation. *Br J Obstet Gynaecol* 1993;100:989–94.

9. North RA, Ferrier C, Long D, Townend K, Kincaid Smith P. Uterine artery Doppler flow velocity waveforms in the second trimester for the prediction of pre-eclampsia and fetal growth retardation. *Obstet Gynecol* 1994;83:378–86.

9 Twin pregnancy

Introduction

Twin pregnancies are associated with significantly increased rates of fetal loss, neonatal loss and neonatal morbidity than singleton pregnancies. Perinatal mortality data collated for the United Kingdom demonstrate a stillbirth rate approximately 2.5–3.0 times that seen in singleton pregnancies and a neonatal loss rate of approximately seven times that seen in singleton pregnancies.[1,2] The adverse outcome of twin pregnancy reflects an increased risk of virtually all obstetric complications, particularly preterm delivery and fetal growth restriction, in addition to specific complications of monochorionic twins.

Classification of twin pregnancy

Twins can be classified by their zygosity (number of fertilised ova – non-identical dizygotic twins or identical monozygotic twins) or by their chorionicity (the number of placentae – dichorionic or monochorionic/one shared placenta). The latter classification is of clinical relevance for three important reasons: (1) it can be determined antenatally, (2) it influences prenatal screening and the management of certain obstetric complications and (3) it predicts the risk of specific complications. Monochorionic twins have a six-fold risk of loss before 24 weeks of gestation[3] and two to three-fold increased risk of stillbirth and early neonatal deaths when compared with dichorionic twins.

EMBRYOLOGY OF MONOCHORIONIC TWIN PREGNANCY

Approximately 30% of twins are identical or monozygotic, of which 70% are monochorionic (Figure 9.1). This occurs when a single fertilised ovum splits into identical twins 3 days after fertilisation. At this point in time, the outer chorion has started to differentiate and so, although embryo division occurs, the resultant fetuses will share an outer chorion (placenta and chorionic membrane). Division of the embryo 8 days post-fertilisation will result in monoamniotic monochorionic twins. Division beyond 13 days occurs during embryonic disk differentiation and these twins will be

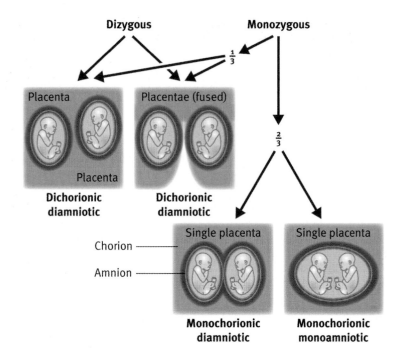

Figure 9.1 The relationship between zygocity and chorionicity

conjoint, monoamniotic monochorionic twins.

Division of an embryo within 3 days of fertilisation will result in identical twins that will each form their own chorion. These twins will be dichorionic diamniotic and will be indistinguishable from same-sex dizygotic (obligatory dichorionic) twins throughout pregnancy.

ANTENATAL DETERMINATION OF CHORIONICITY

Chorionicity can be accurately determined by ultrasound in the first trimester (10–14 weeks of gestation).[4,5] Where two placental masses are identified, the pregnancy is dichorionic. More frequently, an apparent single placental mass exists on ultrasound examination. In this situation, chorionicity can be determined by examination of the inter-twin membrane, where it joins this placental mass. The lambda sign is diagnosed when a tongue of placental tissue (chorionic villi) protrudes into the base of the inter-twin membrane (Figures 9.1 and 9.2). This demonstrates that the inter-twin membrane must represent the fusion of two chorionic in addition to two amniotic membranes and therefore the pregnancy is dichorionic. In a monochorionic pregnancy, the inter-twin

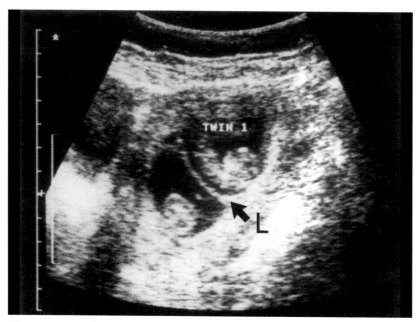

Figure 9.2 The lambda sign; a tongue of placental tissue protrudes into the base of the inter-twin membrane (L) indicating a dichorionic pregnancy

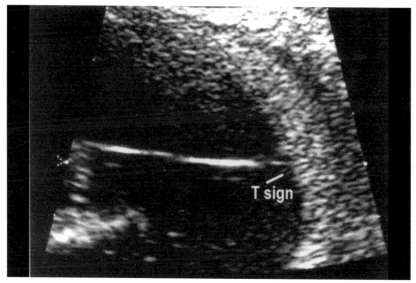

Figure 9.3 The T-sign; the chorionic membrane inserts directly into the placental tissue and indicates a monochorionic twin pregnancy

membrane, a fusion of the two amniotic membranes, cannot obviously contain any chorionic tissue at its base and thus makes a T-sign as it joins the placental mass (Figures 9.1 and 9.3). With advancing gestation, these ultrasound signs are lost and determination of chorionicity in same sex twins may not be possible.

Complications of twin pregnancy: fetal medicine issues

With the possible exception of spontaneous 'unexplained' preterm labour, complications of twin pregnancy requiring fetal medicine input can only be optimally managed if the chorionicity of the pregnancy is known. The remainder of the chapter, subsequent to the discussion of preterm labour, will be subdivided on this basis. Failure to determine chorionicity before 14 weeks of gestation in all booking units should be viewed as substandard care.

Preterm labour

Approximately 25–30% of all twins deliver before 37 weeks of completed gestation. While 89% of all twin deaths occur in this group, the vast majority of perinatal deaths (65%) occur in those pregnancies that deliver before 28 weeks of gestation. Although some twin complications, particularly those affecting monochorionic twins, predispose to premature delivery, 'unexplained' spontaneous preterm labour accounts for the majority of premature births. Uterine overdistension is thought to be an underlying or contributing factor.

MANAGEMENT OF PRETERM LABOUR

Owing to the high risk of twin pregnancies delivering before term, all twin pregnancies presenting with palpable uterine activity should be admitted and 'treated' for preterm labour. Administration of steroids to promote fetal lung maturity should be considered when the pregnancy is less than 35 completed weeks. If there is no evidence of ruptured membranes, tocolytics should also be considered, with the aim of suppressing labour for 48 hours to allow the completion of the steroid therapy. There are no randomised trials that specifically address the use of tocolytics in twin pregnancy and small studies on the use of steroids in twin pregnancies have not demonstrated a significant neonatal benefit in this population. However, the rationale for the use of both these therapies has been extrapolated from extensive studies of singleton pregnancies and seems reasonable.[6] The same doses of treatment should be given in twin as in singleton pregnancy.

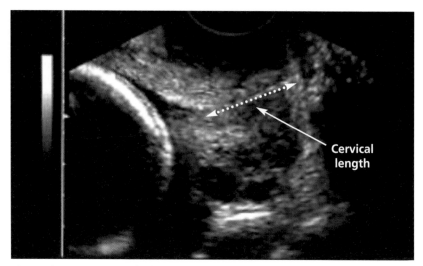

Figure 9.4 Transvaginal ultrasound assessment of cervical length

PREDICTION OF PRETERM LABOUR IN ASYMPTOMATIC TWIN PREGNANCIES

It would be useful to identify those twin pregnancies at highest risk of spontaneous preterm birth before the onset of symptoms, to allow greater time for interventions such as *in utero* transfer, steroids and possible preventative therapies. A number of studies have investigated the predictive role of two potential markers of preterm delivery in asymptomatic twin populations: fetal fibronectin detection in the cervicovaginal secretions and a short cervical length as measured by transvaginal ultrasound. Fetal fibronectin performs inconsistently across studies and therefore does not appear to be a useful test. In contrast, transvaginal ultrasound assessment of cervical length (Figure 9.4) does appear to be a potentially useful predictive test. The majority of studies have suggested that a cervical length of 25 mm or less between 18 and 24 weeks of gestation has moderate value (likelihood ratio close to 5) as a positive screening test for preterm labour.[7,8]

PREVENTION OF SPONTANEOUS PRETERM BIRTH IN TWIN PREGNANCIES

At present there is no proven effective therapy to prevent or delay delivery in twin pregnancies destined to deliver before term. In singleton pregnancies, progesterone therapy in the form of intramuscular 17-hydroxy-progesterone-caproate or vaginal natural progesterone has been demonstrated to reduce the incidence of spontaneous preterm birth in populations at high risk of preterm birth (those with a previous history of preterm birth or with short cervical length on transvaginal ultrasound). Disappointingly in twin gestations, two large studies have not demonstrated a benefit of progesterone therapy to reduce the incidence of preterm birth in general asymptomatic populations.[9,10] A number of further studies are in progress or proposed and the results of these are awaited. A study of the value of progesterone therapy in twin gestations with short cervical length would be of particular interest.

Cervical cerclage does not appear to be a useful measure to prevent preterm birth in twin pregnancies. A randomised study of cervical cerclage in twin pregnancies with a short cervical length demonstrated increased preterm delivery and neonatal loss rates in the cohort randomised to cerclage rather than conservative therapy.[11]

Dichorionic twin pregnancy complications

FETAL STRUCTURAL ABNORMALITIES

Dichorionic twins may or may not have a slightly increased incidence of structural abnormalities than singletons. Robust clinical data are not available. A small increase in incidence could occur from the contribution of the monozygotic dichorionic twin pairs and the pathology of embryo division (see later). The mother has thus, by simple arithmetic, at least a two-fold risk of carrying a fetus with a structural abnormality than if she were carrying a singleton. When diagnosed, the vast majority of fetal abnormalities affect only one twin. In dichorionic twin pregnancies, feticide of a severely anomalous twin can be performed as it is performed in singleton pregnancies, by ultrasound-guided intracardiac injection of potassium chloride. When performed before 18–20 weeks of gestation, there is an approximate 5–9% risk of loss of the healthy co-twin in this 'selective' termination of pregnancy. The risk of loss is highest at the more advanced gestations.[12]

FETAL KARYOTYPE ABNORMALITIES

Since many twin pregnancies occur in older mothers, chromosome abnormalities such as trisomy 21 are not uncommon. As the majority of dichorionic twin pregnancies are dizygous, the pregnancy will have approximately double the maternal age-related risk of carrying at least one fetus with a trisomy.

Second-trimester biochemical screening to calculate risks for trisomy 21 in twin pregnancies is fraught with difficulty and is therefore not offered in the majority of maternity units. First-trimester ultrasound measurements of nuchal translucency in twin pregnancies have been reported.[13]

The test appears to be as reliable in dichorionic twins as in a singleton pregnancy, with a low false-positive rate.

If indicated, karyotyping of both fetuses must be performed in dichorionic twin pregnancies. Most units offer second-trimester amniocentesis and will use more than one needle insertion to ensure accurate uncontaminated sampling of each sac. Chorionic villus sampling is subject to technical difficulties. It may be difficult to access one placenta if they are lying separately or it may be difficult to ensure that both placentas have been sampled if they lie together. Centres that have expertise in performing these diagnostic tests in twin pregnancies report loss rates similar to those seen in singleton pregnancies. Before either diagnostic test is performed, strict mapping of placental sites and fetal characteristics (anomaly or sex) is required to ensure that selective feticide can be appropriately targeted if it is subsequently requested. Confirmatory karyotyping at feticide is good practice.

FETAL GROWTH RESTRICTION

Abdominal palpation is not reliable for monitoring fetal growth in multiple pregnancies. Serial ultrasound should be performed to measure fetal abdominal circumferences, although repeated studies have confirmed that ultrasound may underestimate or overestimate fetal weight by as much as 10%, a similar margin of error as in singleton pregnancies.

A significant difference in the growth of one twin compared with the other is seen in 12% of pregnancies and approximately 30% of twins are small for gestational age. Dizygotic twins, having completely distinct genetic material, will have different growth potentials and may demonstrate discordant growth patterns while being healthy. Alternatively, both twins may be growth-restricted and may show no growth discordance. For these reasons, assessment of liquor volumes should be performed, with determination of growth velocity, to detect those fetuses which, irrespective of size, are compromised *in utero*.

If suspected, fetal growth restriction requires increased surveillance of fetal wellbeing with Doppler monitoring and cardiotocography, so that delivery can be optimally timed. In dichorionic pregnancies, severe growth restriction of one twin at a very preterm gestation may be best managed conservatively in the interest of the larger twin: allowing a possible single intrauterine death rather than planned very premature delivery of both twins.

INTRAUTERINE DEATH OF ONE TWIN

During the first trimester, a significant number of twin pregnancies miscarry completely and up to 30% of all pregnancies diagnosed as twins continue as a singleton pregnancy following the demise of one twin. Intrauterine death of one twin in the late second or third trimester occurs in approximately 2% of dichorionic pregnancies. A number will be due to fetal growth restriction or cord accidents but frequently no specific cause of death can be identified antenatally or at postmortem examination. The main risk to the surviving twin is of premature delivery. The death of one twin *in utero* will usually stimulate uterine activity and most pregnancies will deliver within 3 weeks of the death occurring.

Retention of dead fetal material *in utero* is associated with the development of maternal coagulation problems in singleton pregnancies. This appears to be considerably less likely in twin pregnancies with a single intrauterine fetal death. Nevertheless, it may be prudent to monitor maternal coagulatory and infective parameters at least once weekly in this scenario.

Where the single intrauterine fetal death occurs beyond 34 weeks of gestation, delivery of the surviving twin should be planned. In advance of delivery, most would advocate administration of antenatal steroids and, if fetal monitoring were satisfactory, conservative management of the pregnancy until 34 weeks of gestation. While there is no clear evidence that mode of delivery affects the outcome of the surviving twin, many of these pregnancies are delivered by caesarean section.

Monochorionic twin pregnancy complications

The embryology of monochorionic twins (late division) places them at high risk of complications. The shared monochorionic placenta is either the cause of complications or confounds the risk of these complications. In virtually all monochorionic placentas, there is a shared central portion in which there exists a number of arterial to venous anastomoses, venous to venous anastomoses and arterial to arterial anastomoses between the two fetoplacental circulations. Pathology is dictated by the presence, type and relative numbers of these anastomoses. As will soon be evident, the spectre of a single intrauterine death in any complication affecting monochorionic twins strongly influences the fetal medicine approach to management.

SINGLE INTRAUTERINE FETAL DEATH

The death of one monochorionic twin *in utero* carries with it severe risks to the co-twin, as a direct result of the vascular anastomoses between the two fetoplacental circulations. Upon death, the vascular tone of a fetus is lost and its fetoplacental vascular volume expands, draining the fetoplacental volume of the co-twin. The co-twin is therefore at risk of severe acute hypotension and organ hypoxia. Toxic thromboplastins may also be released from the dead twin tissue and may pass through the joint circulation into the co-twin, compounding organ damage. It is estimated that there is a 30% risk of co-twin death or, if this twin survives, a 20% risk of severe neurological damage.[14]

Typically, diagnosis of single intrauterine fetal death occurs in an unknown time period after the event. Early delivery of the survivor is not indicated, as any pathology will have occurred; premature delivery may confound the risk of adverse outcome. The fetus can be monitored by ultrasound for overt neurological damage such as hydrocephalus. Earlier evidence of neurological damage may be possible by magnetic resonance imaging. Leukomalacia or brain atrophy of the surviving twin may be seen 3 weeks after the death of the other.[15] In these circumstances, termination of pregnancy is an option for the parents. In the absence of these signs, the neurological outcome of the survivor is difficult to predict.

If the diagnosis of single intrauterine fetal death occurs within 48 hours of the event, immediate intrauterine transfusion to 'restore' the circulating volume of the survivor and attempt to reduce the risk of neurological morbidity has been attempted. However, the success of such intervention is not proven and assessment is continuing in specialised centres.

FETAL STRUCTURAL ABNORMALITIES

Monochorionic twins have an increased risk of structural abnormality over dichorionic twins. The process of embryo division appears to be intrinsically teratogenic. Change may occur either because embryo division results in two uneven cell masses or embryo division occurs after certain cells have differentiated their polarity. Anomalies of the heart, such as a non-symmetrical organ, are common, supporting the later mechanism. Neural tube abnormalities are also prevalent. Anomalies of the cerebral cortex, kidneys and gut also occur. The aetiology of the latter may reflect a destructive influence; that is, acute hypoxia owing to fluxes in interfetal cardiovascular perfusion. The incidence of structural anomalies increases with the lateness of embryo division. The congenital anomaly rate is approximately three to four-fold higher in monochorionic diamniotic pregnancies than in dichorionic or singleton pregnancies, approximately 20–25% in monochorionic monoamniotic twins and, in conjoint twins, structural anomalies of even unshared organs occurs in up to 80% of cases.

In monochorionic diamniotic twins, the structural abnormality affects only one twin in 80% of cases . In this situation, management options and parental counselling are difficult. Paradoxically, fetal anomalies that are likely to be nonviable may not be best managed conservatively. Severe structural anomalies place a fetus at increased risk of intrauterine death, with its resultant risks to the co-twin. Additionally, anomalies such as anencephaly or diaphragmatic hernia are typically complicated by polyhydramnios and place the co-twin at risk of severe preterm delivery owing to uterine distension.

Selective termination of pregnancy by intracardiac potassium chloride cannot be used, as it can in dichorionic twin pregnancies, owing to the vascular anastomoses between the two fetoplacental circulations. Cord occlusive techniques by interstitial laser (less than 20 weeks of gestation), bipolar diathermy (17–25 weeks of gestation) or ligation (advanced gestation) are the only 'selective' option for termination in mono-chorionic twin pregnancies.[15,16] These techniques can only be attempted in a small number of highly specialised fetal medicine units. Owing to their relatively invasive nature, they carry a significant risk of membrane rupture (10–30%) and loss of the structurally normal twin.

FETAL KARYOTYPE ABNORMALITIES

As monochorionic twin pregnancies arise from division of a single fertilised oocyte, the maternal risk of pregnancy being complicated by a trisomy of both fetuses is the same as the age-related risk of a singleton pregnancy. Nuchal translucency measurements perform less accurately as a predictor of karyotype abnormalities in monochorionic compared with dichorionic twins. This is because large nuchal measurements are more commonly observed in karyotypically normal monochorionic twins. A large nuchal translucency may reflect an underlying tendency to later development of twin–twin transfusion syndrome or a cardiac structural anomaly. Nevertheless, nuchal measurements remain a useful addition to maternal age in the calculation of risk of karyotype abnormality. An averaged measurement appears to act as the best screening test for trisomy.[17]

In general, following a high-risk screening result, sampling of only one pool of amniotic fluid, placenta or fetus is performed in monochorionic twin pregnancies, as the genetic material is almost always identical in both twins. Discordant karyotype abnormalities can rarely occur, owing to post-zygotic mutations or loss of genetic material (that is, XO with XX or XY 'identical' twin) and so the need to sample both twins should be considered when discordant structural anomalies are seen.

FETAL GROWTH RESTRICTION

The underlying pathophysiology of fetal growth restriction may be modified in monochorionic twins as a result of the inter-twin vascular anastomoses within the monochorionic placenta. A moderate degree of placental insufficiency related to one twin may be exaggerated by a degree of blood donation from that fetoplacental circulation to that of the co-twin, producing severe growth restriction. Alternatively, the twin with placental insufficiency may be 'donated' blood and may demonstrate normal growth. The existence of the placental vascular anastomoses also affects the resistance of blood flow through the umbilical cord vessels, making Doppler studies less reliable. Detection and monitoring of placental insufficiency is therefore problematic.

The consequences of growth restriction are also far greater in monochorionic pregnancies, as one twin's viability is directly linked to the other's via their shared placental vasculature. There is therefore a much lower threshold for planned preterm delivery in a monochorionic twin pregnancy demonstrating selective growth restriction than in a dichorionic twin pregnancy, to avoid the death of one twin. The decision to deliver versus trying to stretch out conservative management can be agonising at extremely preterm gestations.

If a single intrauterine fetal death is anticipated before a viable gestation, selective feticide by a cord occlusive technique may be considered by specialised centres. To date, this has not been proven to be beneficial for the co-twin's outcome. A randomised clinical trial comparing conservative management with laser ablation therapy of placental anastomosing vessels (as in twin–twin transfusion syndrome) is currently being conducted in monochorionic twin pregnancies complicated by severe growth restriction of one fetus. This study will assess whether laser therapy to 'un-link' the two fetal circulations and so allow each fetus to 'independently' take its chances with advancing gestation, would be beneficial to the neonatal outcome of either or both twins.

Specific complications of monochorionic twins

TWIN–TWIN TRANSFUSION SYNDROME

Twin–twin transfusion syndrome complicates 10–15% of monochorionic twins. The pathological condition occurs as the result of a net transfer of blood from one 'donor' twin to the other 'recipient' twin through unidirectional arterial to venous anastomoses within the placenta (Figure 9.5). The lack of a bidirectional arterial-to-arterial anastomosis, a potential compensatory redistribution channel, is also believed to contribute to the pathological state.[18–20] The unbalanced sharing of blood results in a volume overloaded 'recipient' twin and a hypovolaemic 'donor' twin. The recipient develops polyhydramnios (polyuria) (Figure 9.6) and may progress to congestive cardiac failure, hydrops and death. The polyhydramnios may cause rapid uterine expansion and may precipitate labour and delivery as early as 16–24 weeks of gestation. The 'donor' redistributes blood flow to vital organs, resulting in growth restriction and oligohydramnios (reduced renal perfusion). This twin is also at risk of cardiac (high-output) failure and death. The severity and prognosis of twin–twin transfusion syndrome can be staged by ultrasound (Table 9.1);[21] however,

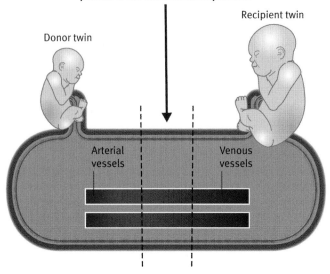

Arterial to venous anastomoses within the shared portion of the monochorionic placenta

Donor twin

Recipient twin

Arterial vessels

Venous vessels

Figure 9.5 Proposed mechanism for the development of twin–twin transfusion syndrome

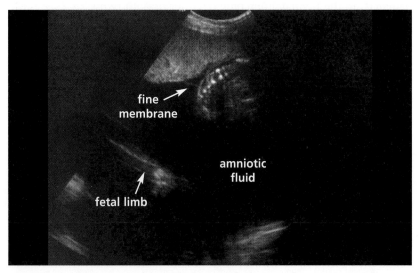

fine membrane

amniotic fluid

fetal limb

Figure 9.6 Ultrasound of twin–twin transfusion syndrome; the small 'donor' twin appears stuck to the placenta by the closely applied membrane, reflecting severe oligohydramnios in its amniotic sac; the recipient twin is surrounded by polyhydramnios

Table 9.1   Quintero staging of twin–twin transfusion syndrome (TTTS)[21]

Quintero stage	Ultrasound findings[a]
I	Polyhydramnios (> 8 cm maximal vertical pocket [MVP] on one side of dividing amniotic membranes and oligohydramnios (< 2 cm MVP) on the other side[b]
II	Bladder of the donor twin not visible (empty)
III	Abnormal arterial or venous Doppler in either twin[c]
IV	Hydrops fetalis (cardiac failure) of either twin
V	Intrauterine demise of one or both twins

[a] This is an ultrasound-derived assessment of disease severity
[b] These are the minimal diagnostic criteria for TTTS and will be present at each stage
[c] The donor twin can typically develop absent end-diastolic flow in the umbilical artery, a sign of increased vascular resistance/reduced placental perfusion; the recipient can develop a reversed α-wave in the ductus venosus, a sign of cardiac overload

there is an 80–95% overall fetal loss rate without intervention.

The condition is also associated with a high morbidity rate in any liveborn infants. Even with specialised fetal medicine intervention, up to 15% of survivors have serious neurological morbidity, such as cerebral palsy. Heart valve damage is identified in 12% of 'recipient' twins at birth. Renal and gastrointestinal complications may also occur.

A number of therapies have been attempted to improve the outcome of this condition. Only two are currently considered useful: serial amniodrainage or laser ablation therapy of the causative placental vascular anastomoses. Amniodrainage, the removal of large volumes (2–3 litres) of amniotic fluid from the recipient's sac to achieve a normal volume, acts to reduce the distension of the uterus and so reduces the risk of spontaneous preterm labour or miscarriage. It requires to be repeated at regular intervals as the underlying pathological process continues.

Laser therapy is performed under regional or local anaesthesia. Under ultrasound guidance, a cannula and 2–3 mm fetoscope is inserted into the recipient's amniotic sac. This allows direct visualisation of the vessels on the fetal surface of the placenta. The anastomosing vessels are then selectively coagulated using a laser fibre. Excess amniotic fluid is removed from the recipient's sac before the cannula is removed. Ideally, after completion of the therapy, the twins will be vascularly disconnected from each other. This therapy therefore seeks to correct the underlying pathophysiology of this condition.

There are a number of non-randomised comparable series of laser therapy and amnioreduction. These studies have suggested improved fetal outcomes with laser therapy, especially in advanced-stage disease.[22–24] The first randomised controlled trial comparing laser ablation with amnioreduction also suggested that laser therapy was the most effective intervention (70% survival compared with 50% survival with amnioreduction).[25] Laser therapy was also associated with a lower rate of significant neurological morbidity in surviving twins than amnioreduction (5% compared with 15%).[25] A further randomised control trial was halted very prematurely in recruitment when laser therapy appeared to perform poorly compared with amnioreduction in stage III/IV disease.[26] The finding of this study has been questioned and laser therapy is still generally considered the optimal therapy for advanced-stage disease. It should be provided in a specialised centre for fetal therapy.[27]

Twin–twin transfusion can occur as early as 16 weeks of gestation. Intervention is required typically by 21–22 weeks of gestation so timely recognition of this condition is required to influence outcome. Optimal ultrasound surveillance can be performed by abdominal circumference estimations and measurement of the maximal depth of liquor on each side of the fused amniotic membranes at fortnightly intervals from 14 weeks of gestation.

TWIN REVERSED ARTERIAL PERFUSION SEQUENCE

On rare occasions (approximately 1% of monochorionic twins) one normal twin will develop with an abnormal twin that has no independent cardiac activity but is perfused by the normal twin. The initial pathology of the condition is uncertain; perhaps the acardiac twin was anomalous from conception or was initially normally formed but died *in utero*. Thereafter, the pathological state depends on the presence of large interfetal arterial to arterial anastomoses within the monochorionic placenta. These effect continued perfusion and 'growth' of the anomalous or dead twin by the circulatory output of the normal twin.

Normally, oxygenated blood originating from the placenta enters a fetus through its umbilical artery, the majority of which is then shunted through the ductus venosus to preferentially oxygenate the upper fetal structures, the brain and heart. In twin reversed arterial perfusion (TRAP) sequence, the anomalous or dead twin is perfused in a reverse manner via its artery. The blood is poorly oxygenated, having originated from the other 'pump' twin. This poorly oxygenated blood also perfuses the lower part of the fetus first. The upper fetal structures, including the heart, undergo secondary atrophy and the resultant 'twin' has been described as an 'acardiac monster' (Figure 9.7a,b).

There is a 50–75% incidence of mortality in the 'pump' twin, owing to intrauterine cardiac failure and polyhydramnios-induced preterm delivery. The risk of loss of the pump twin increases if the relative size of

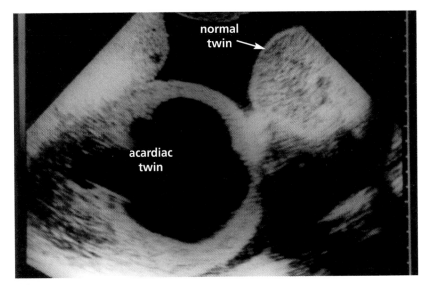

(a)

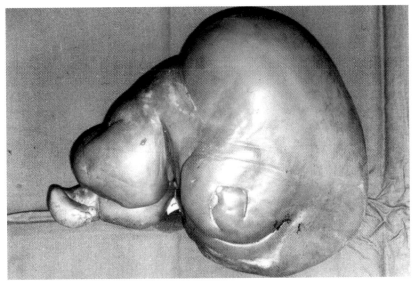

(b)

Figure 9.7 Twin reverse arterial perfusion sequence: (a) transabdominal ultrasound image of a large acardiac twin in transverse section at 28 weeks of gestation; an abdominal cross-section of the normal twin is also seen in this image illustrating the massive size discrepancy; (b) the acardiac twin shown in Figure 9.7a after delivery three weeks later

the acardiac twin is greater than 50% of the pump twin. Venous Doppler ultrasound can be used to survey the pump twin for signs of cardiac failure and to facilitate optimal delivery timing. If signs of cardiac failure are evident before 24 weeks of gestation, cord occlusion of the acardiac twin has been used with success (up to 80% survival of the pump twin) in specialised centres.[28]

MONOAMNIOTIC TWINS

Monoamniotic twins occur in less than 1–2% of twin pregnancies. These twins share a single amniotic sac and are therefore at risk of cord entanglement *in utero*. The twins also have an increased incidence of structural abnormal-ities. Owing to these complications, the twins have risk of mortality of approximately 20–40%.

The outcome can be improved by intensive cardiotocography monitoring once the twins reach viability. The recommended frequency of fetal heart rate monitoring varies between once weekly to three times daily in reported series. Antenatal corticosteroids are usually prescribed to attain fetal lung maturity between 24 and 28 weeks of gestation. Delivery is indicated if cord compression is subsequently diagnosed. Otherwise, as fetal death can occur abruptly in spite of recent reassuring fetal monitoring, delivery is electively planned for 32 weeks of gestation when reasonable fetal maturity has been reached. Delivery should be performed by caesarean section, as the risk of a cord accident is particularly high during labour.

Oligohydramnios induced by non-steroidal anti-inflammatory drugs (NSAIDs) has been suggested as a management strategy to 'splint' and reduce fetal movement to reduce the risks of cord accident and fetal death. A study of the NSAID sulindac in addition to intensive monitoring and delivery at 32 weeks of gestation demonstrated excellent outcomes.[29] However, this treatment has not been proven to improve fetal outcome as an independent variable. Cord entanglement is present in virtually all cases by an early gestation and, in theory, oligohydramnios may increase the risk of cord accident by compression forces.

CONJOINT TWINS

Conjoint twins are another rare complication of monochorionic twins, with an incidence of approximately 1/1000 twin pregnancies. The embryology of their formation is not understood. Incomplete division of the embryonic disk or fusions of embryos at symmetrical developmental axes are proposed theories.

Conjoint twins are most readily diagnosed in the first trimester (Figure 9.8). They are subsequently described according to their main site of fusion. The most common subtypes of conjoint twins consist of those

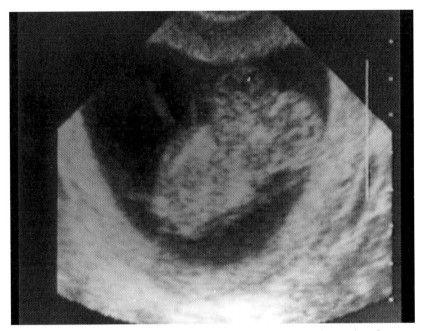

Figure 9.8 Transvaginal ultrasound of conjoint twins at 10 weeks of gestation; the twins were joined at the chest and abdomen but two independent heartbeats were identified

joined at the chest (thoracopagus) or chest and abdomen. Those joined only at the abdomen (omphalopagus) are less common. Rare presentations include those joined at the pelvis (ishiopagus) and cranium (craniopagus). Structural abnormalities of internal organs occur in virtually all cases. Shared cardiac structures, a shared common bile duct and shared posterior cerebral structures have extremely poor prognoses. Up to 50% of conjoint twins die *in utero*. Of those that survive birth, 30% will not be suitable for surgery and will die in the early neonatal period. In cases selected for surgery, there is a 50% infant survival rate in the short term.[30]

Parents require accurate counselling about fetal outcomes and the chances of separation. Termination of pregnancy is commonly requested. If the pregnancy continues, detailed structural survey of the twins is required to allow forward planning of any appropriate surgery. Delivery, by caesarean section, should be performed at a tertiary unit with appropriate obstetric, neonatal and paediatric staff available. The uterine incision is likely to be significant in size and may require vertical extension. This will have adverse implications for the delivery and outcome of future pregnancies.

Table 9.2 Ultrasound surveillance schedule for twin pregnancy

Gestation (weeks)	Ultrasound assessment	
	Dichorionic twins	Monochorionic twins
10–14	Chorionicity, NT screen	Chorionicity, NT screen
14–24		Survey for TTTS (AC and LV fortnightly)[a]
18	Anomaly scan	Anomaly scan
20–22		Fetal ECHO
24–40	Growth (2–4 week intervals)[a]	Growth (fortnightly)[a]

[a] abnormal findings will require more intensive surveillance; AC = abdominal circumference, LV = liquor volume (maximal depth of largest pool on each side of the inter-twin membrane); NT = nuchal translucency measurement; TTTS = twin–twin transfusion syndrome

Summary

The chorionicity of a twin pregnancy should be determined by ultrasound before 14 weeks of gestation. Care of twin pregnancies should be provided at a specialist-led multiple pregnancy clinic. Frequent ultrasound assessments underpin effective screening surveillance of twin fetuses for anomaly, growth and complications (Table 9.2). Monochorionic twins discordant for fetal anomalies, affected by twin–twin transfusion syndrome, severe fetal growth restriction of one twin or single-twin demise should be referred to the regional fetal medicine centre with recourse to specialist expertise.

References

1. Confidential Enquiries into Maternal and Child Health. *Perinatal Mortality 2007: United Kingdom*. London: CEMACH; 2009 [www.cmace.org.uk/getattachment/1d2c0ebc-d2aa-4131-98ed-56bf8269e529/Perinatal-Mortality-2007.aspx].

2. NHS Quality Improvement Scotland. Scottish Programme for Clinical Effectiveness in Reproductive Health. *Scottish Perinatal and Infant Mortality and Morbidity Report 2008*. Edinburgh: NHS QIS; 2010 [www.nhshealthquality.org/nhsqis/7491.html].

3. Sebire N, Snijders R, Hughes K, Sepulveda W, Nicolaides KH. The hidden morbidity of monochorionic twin pregnancies. *Br J Obstet Gynaecol* 1997;104:1203–7.

4. Finberg HJ. The 'twin-peak' sign: reliable evidence of dichorionic twinning. *J Ultrasound Med* 1992;11:571–7.

5. Sepulveda W, Seibre NJ, Hughes K, Odibo A, Nicolaides KH. The lambda sign at 10–14 weeks gestation as a predictor of chorionicity in twin pregnancies. *Ultrasound Obstet Gynaecol* 1996;7:421–3.

6. Royal College of Obstetricians and Gynaecologists. *Antenatal Corticosteroids to Prevent Respiratory Distress Syndrome*. London: RCOG; 2004 [www.rcog.org.uk/womens-health/clinical-guidance/antenatal-corticosteroids-prevent-respiratory-distress-syndrome-gree].

7. Skentou C, Souka AP, To MS, Liao AW, Nicolaides KH. Prediction of preterm delivery in twins by cervical assessment at 23 weeks. *Ultrasound Obstet Gynecol* 2001;17:7–10.

8. Gibson JL, Macara LM, Owen P, Young D, Macauley J, Mackenzie F. Prediction of preterm delivery in twin pregnancy: a prospective, observational study of cervical length and fetal fibronectin testing. *Ultrasound Obstet Gynecol* 2004;23:561–6.

9. Rouse DJ, Caritis SN, Peaceman AM, Sciscione A, Thom EA, Spong CY, *et al*. A trial of 17 alpha-hydroxyprogesterone caproate to prevent prematurity in twins. *N Engl J Med* 2007;357:454–61.

10. Norman J, Mackenzie F, Owen P, Mactier H, Hanretty K, Cooper S, *et al*. Progesterone for the prevention of premature birth in twin pregnancy (STOPPIT): a randomized, double-blind, placebo-controlled study and meta-analysis. *Lancet* 2009;373:2034–40.

11. Berghella V, Obido AO, To MS, Rust OA, Althiusius SM. Cerclage for short cervix on ultrasound: meta-analysis of trials using individual patient-level data. *Obstet Gynecol* 2005;106:181-9.

12. Evans MI, Goldberg JD, Horenstein J, Wapner RJ, Ayoub MA, Sone J, *et al*. Selective termination for structural, chromosomal, and Mendelian anomalies: international experience. *Am J Obstet Gynecol* 1999;181:893–7.

13. Sebire NJ, Snijders RJM, Hughes K, Sepulveda W, Nicolaides KH. Screening for trisomy 21 in twin pregnancies by maternal age and fetal nuchal translucency at 10–14 weeks of gestation. *Br J Obstet Gynaecol* 1996;103:999–1003.

14. Pharoah PO, Adi Y. Consequences of *in-utero* death in a twin pregnancy. *Lancet* 2000;355:1597–602.

15. Lewi L, Van Schoubroeck D, Gratacos E, Witters I, Timmerman D, Deprest J. Monochorionic diamniotic twins: complications and management. *Curr Opin Obstet Gynecol* 2003;15:177–94.

16. Chmait RH, Quintero RA. Operative fetoscopy in complicated monochorionic twins: current status and future direction. *Curr Opin Obstet Gynecol* 2008;20:169–74.

17. Vandecruys H, Faiola S, Auer M, Sebire N, Nicolaides KH. Screening for trisomy 21 in monochorionic twins by measurement of the fetal nuchal translucency thickness. *Ultrasound Obstet Gynecol* 2005;25:551–3.

18. Diehl W, Hecher K, Zikulnig L, Vetter M, Hackeloer BJ. Placental vascular anastomoses visualised during fetoscopic laser surgery in severe mid-trimester twin-twin transfusion syndrome. *Placenta* 2001;22:876–81.

19. Umur A, van Gemert MJC, Nikkels PGJ, Ross MG. Monochorionic twins and twin–twin transfusion syndrome: the protective role of arterio-arterial anastomoses. *Placenta* 2002;23:201–9.

20. Wee LY, Fisk N. The twin–twin transfusion syndrome. *Semin Neonatal* 2002;7:187–202.

21. Quintero RA, Morales WJ, Allen MH, Bornick PW, Johnson PK, Kruger M. Staging of twin–twin transfusion syndrome. *J Perinatol* 1999;19:550–5.

22. Hecher K, Plath H, Bregenzer T, Hasmann M, Hackeloer BJ. Endoscopic laser surgery versus serial amniocentesis in the treatment of severe twin–twin transfusion syndrome. *Am J Obstet Gynecol* 1999;180:717–24.

23. Ville Y, Hyett J, Hecher K, Nicolaides K. Preliminary experience with endoscopic laser therapy for severe twin–twin transfusion syndrome. *N Engl J Med* 1995;332:224–7.

24. Quintero RA, Dickinson JE, Morales WJ, Bornick PW, Bermundez C, Cincotta R, *et al*. Stage-based treatment of twin-to-twin transfusion syndrome. *Am J Obstet Gynecol* 2003;188:1333–40.

25. Senat MV, Deprest J, Boulvain M, Paupe A, Winer N, Ville Y. Endoscopic laser surgery versus serial amnioreduction for severe twin-to-twin transfusion syndrome. *N Eng J Med* 2004;351:36–44.

26. Crombleholme TM, Shera D, Lee H, Johnson M, D'Alton M, Porter F, *et al*. A prospective, randomized, multicenter trial of amnioreduction vs. selective fetoscopic laser photocoagulation for the treatment of severe twin-twin transfusion syndrome. *Am J Obstet Gynecol* 2007;197:e391–9.

27. National Institute for Health and Clinical Excellence. *Intrauterine Laser Ablation of Placental Vessels for the Treatment of Twin-to-Twin Transfusion Syndrome.* Interventional Procedure Guidance 198. London: NICE; 2006 [www.nice.org.uk/IPG198].

28. Quintero RA, Chmait RH, Murakoshi T, Barigyne O, Chappell L, Fisk N. Surgical management of twin reversed arterial perfusion sequence. *Am J Obstet Gynecol* 2006;194:982–91.

29. Pasquini L, Wimalasundera RC, Fichera A, Barigye O, Chappell L, Fisk NM. High perinatal survival in monoamniotic twins managed by prophylactic sulindac, intensive ultrasound surveillance, and cesarean delivery at 32 weeks' gestation. *Ultrasound Obstet Gynecol* 2006;28:681–7.

30. Spitz L, Kiely EM. Experience in the management of conjoint twins. *Br J Surg* 2002;89:1188–92.

10 Fetal infection

Introduction

There are many infections that have the potential to pose risk to the fetus and neonate. When considering congenital infection, it is important to take account of a number of factors. Who is at risk of infection and what is the risk of transmission to the fetus? What is the best method of diagnosing fetal infection and, if the fetus is infected, can we predict whether or not it is affected and if so to what extent? Is there anything that can be done to prevent or treat fetal infection? This chapter addresses these questions for some of the infections that are associated with adverse outcome in pregnancy.

Cytomegalovirus

Cytomegalovirus (CMV) is the leading cause of congenital viral infection and is, as a result, a common cause of sensorineural deafness and mental restriction. It is found in all geographical locations. In industrialised countries, approximately 50% of women are immune to CMV at the outset of pregnancy.

CMV is a member of the herpes family. A feature of this family of viruses, which includes herpes simplex, varicella zoster and Ebstein Barr virus, is that after primary infection the virus remains alive but usually dormant within the host's body. There is therefore the potential for reactivation of infection at a time distant from the primary infection.[1]

Primary infection occurs in 1–2 % of pregnancies and is responsible for approximately two-thirds of the cases of congenital CMV. Recurrent infection accounts for the remaining one-third of cases of congenital CMV. The vertical transmission rate is 20–40% following primary infection and approximately 1% following recurrent infection. While previous infection is protective against congenital infection, it does not prevent it completely and it has been estimated that maternal immunity reduces the risk of congenital CMV in future pregnancies by 69%.[2]

Recurrent infection can occur as a result of reactivation of latent virus or reinfection by a different virus strain. The relative importance of these two mechanisms remains undetermined. Serological testing cannot differentiate these two mechanisms of recurrent infection. Clinical symptoms are less common with recurrent infection but it is recognised that severe disease can occur.[2]

The virus has been isolated in saliva, blood, urine, faeces, semen, vaginal fluids, breast milk and tears. Viral spread is via direct contact. The incubation period is 2–3 weeks. The risk of seroconversion in pregnancy is lowest in women of high socio-economic status or with good personal hygiene.

DIAGNOSIS

Maternal CMV infection is usually asymptomatic, although some women may experience a flu-like illness with fever and mild hepatitis. Maternal serology is most helpful when the woman's prepregnancy CMV status is known. The identification of CMV-specific immunoglobulin G (IgG) antibodies in a woman previously known to be seronegative for CMV indicates primary infection in the current pregnancy. The presence of both IgG and immunoglobulin M (IgM) in a woman of unknown CMV status makes interpretation more difficult, as IgM antibodies can persist in the circulation for up to 18 months. Their presence may therefore indicate infection remote from pregnancy or it may indicate primary or preconceptional infection with CMV.

Preconceptional infection within 6 months of pregnancy still poses a risk of fetal infection. A false positive IgM result can occur in the presence of rheumatoid factor of IgM subclass or as a result of cross-reactivity with other herpes virus infections. IgG avidity testing has been employed to try to differentiate recent and past CMV infection. This relies on the fact that antibodies bind less avidly to antigens in the early stages of infection, in contrast to the chronic stages of infection. A low IgG avidity result suggests recent infection whereas a high avidity result indicates more distant infection.

FETAL INFECTION

The mechanisms involved in vertical transmission remain unclear. The rate of transmission is not significantly influenced by gestational age, in contrast to the outcome of transmission, which will be discussed later. Once primary infection or reactivation of maternal CMV has been established, prenatal diagnosis should be offered to determine the risk of fetal infection. CMV can be detected in fetal blood and amniotic fluid. The virus replicates in the fetal kidney. It takes 5–7 weeks post-fetal infection for a sufficient quantity of virus to be excreted via fetal urine into the amniotic fluid. CMV can be detected in amniotic fluid by culture, polymerase chain reaction (PCR) to detect and quantify CMV-DNA or amplification techniques to identify messenger RNA of specific CMV proteins. The overall sensitivity of

PCR detection of CMV in amniotic fluid ranges from 70–100%.[3] The reliability of testing is greatest when performed at the appropriate time; that is, after 21 weeks of gestation, and at least 6 weeks after maternal infection.[4] Testing of fetal blood for CMV-specific IgM is not recommended because many fetuses do not mount an immune response until later in pregnancy, so there is the risk of a false-negative result. In addition, the procedure-related loss rate is higher. Amniocentesis is the preferred option for prenatal diagnosis of CMV.

If the diagnosis of CMV infection has not been made in the antenatal period, testing must take place within 2 weeks of birth if congenital infection is to be confirmed. After this time, the presence of CMV can be from acquired neonatal infection, which has few, if any, symptoms and complications. The gold-standard for diagnosis is virus isolation in cell culture.

IMPLICATIONS OF FETAL INFECTION

CMV infection leads to enlargement of cells with intranuclear inclusions, which may result in cell death. The organs commonly affected include the brain, liver and placenta. Infection during the first half of pregnancy is associated with more severe fetal disease. Ten to fifteen percent of neonates with primary CMV infection will be symptomatic. Of these, approximately 5% will die and 90% of the survivors will have neurodevelopmental damage including mental restriction, sensorineural deafness and visual impairment.[5] It is impossible to predict accurately the extent of neuro-developmental impairment at birth. In addition, 10–15% of asymptomatic children will develop some degree of deafness and or learning difficulties.

Ultrasound features indicative of symptomatic CMV infection include hyperechogenic bowel, ascites, fetal growth restriction, ventriculomegaly and other brain abnormalities, of which periventricular calcification is a common finding. It is recognised that these ultrasound findings are not specific for CMV infection but are also found in other fetal infections and pathology. There is a correlation between antenatal or neonatal intra-cranial abnormalities and adverse neurodevelopmental outcome. However, a normal antenatal scan does not rule out long-term sequelae.

The most common findings in symptomatic neonates are petechiae and thrombocytopenia (60–80%), hepatosplenomegaly (70%), jaundice (55%), growth restriction (40%) and microcephaly (40%). Microcephaly from birth onwards is the most sensitive predictor of mental restriction.

MANAGEMENT

Once maternal infection is established, amniocentesis should be offered, at the appropriate interval, to determine the risk of fetal infection. Serial scans can be carried out at fortnightly intervals for evidence of the ultrasound features described above. Fetal magnetic resonance imaging may give additional information and should be offered at 32 and 36 weeks of gestation. There is evidence that prenatal ultrasound anomalies and fetal thrombocytopenia are strong and independent predictors of poor fetal outcome.[6] Increasing severity of thrombocytopenia is associated with a poorer prognosis. Establishing the fetal platelet count by cordocentesis could be used as a predictor of adverse outcome in those cases of confirmed fetal infection with normal ultrasound findings.

POTENTIAL THERAPY

The optimal treatment strategy for congenital CMV has yet to be established. At the present time, there is no *in utero* therapy to limit the sequelae of fetal infection. Maternal oral administration of the antiretroviral agent valaciclovir does result in therapeutic drug concentrations in mother and fetus. In addition, it is associated with a decrease in viral load in fetal blood.[7] These are preliminary data and a randomised controlled trial is required to investigate a role for this drug in the antenatal management of fetal CMV infection. Since maternal infections are largely asymptomatic, it is unlikely that targeting drug therapy to reduce vertical transmission will be achievable. Rather, a control on the impact of congenital disease should be the focus.

COUNSELLING

There are a number of uncertainties to be discussed when counselling a woman with confirmed CMV infection in pregnancy, for the following reasons:

- maternal infection does not result in fetal infection in the majority of cases
- there is a necessary time lag between maternal infection and embarking upon prenatal diagnosis of fetal infection
- fetal infection does not mean that the fetus is affected: only 10–15% of infected babies are symptomatic at birth
- ultrasound features that may indicate an affected baby take a number of weeks to develop
- antenatal detection of a symptomatic fetus is indicative of long-term sequelae
- a normal ultrasound scan does not rule out an affected baby: abnormalities are observed in less than 50% of the infected fetuses
- asymptomatic babies can also have long-term sequelae in 10–15% of cases
- the overall risk of an adverse fetal or neonatal outcome following primary maternal CMV infection is approximately 7–10%.

ROUTINE SCREENING FOR CMV

Routine screening for CMV remains a controversial area and, although CMV is an important health problem, other World Health Organization criteria for an effective screening programme cannot be met. As discussed above, interpretation of maternal CMV serology can be complex. The presence of IgM does not necessarily indicate recent infection, owing to the length of time that IgM can persist in the circulation. Avidity testing can be helpful but it is not considered by all laboratories to be accurate and reliable. There is no vaccine available to prevent CMV infection and, as yet, no effective treatment to prevent the long-term sequelae of infection. Preconceptional knowledge that a woman is seronegative for CMV would, however, be useful in the event of suspected CMV infection during pregnancy, as this would enable differentiation between primary and secondary infection.

Toxoplasmosis

Toxoplasmosis gondii is an obligate intracellular protozoan parasite. There are two phases to its life cycle.[8] The sexual phase takes place only in cats (definitive host), whereas the asexual phase can take place in any warm-blooded animal (intermediate host: mammals or birds). Tissue cysts contain bradyzoites, the slowly replicating form of the parasite. Feline ingestion of tissue cysts (carnivorism) leads to release of the parasites and infection of epithelial cells of the cat's small intestine. Sexual replication takes place within the small intestine resulting in the formation of oocysts which are then excreted in cat faeces into the environment. Three to five days later the oocysts undergo sporolation, producing highly infectious sporozoites that can survive in the environment for a number of years. Following ingestion by an intermediate host, such as a mouse or human, the sporozoites undergo differentiation to tachyzoites, which are responsible for acute infection. At this point in the life cycle, congenital transmission to the fetus can occur. In many intermediate hosts a chronic phase of infection will ensue, as the tachyzoite transforms to the slowly replicating bradyzoite, which is contained within tissue cysts. Ingestion of a chronically infected intermediate host by a cat will propagate the continuing cycle (Figure 10.1).

T. *gondii* infection occurs most frequently following ingestion of raw or undercooked meats, ingestion of infected food, water or contaminated soil. Toxoplasmosis infection in humans is frequently asymptomatic or subclinical. Following an incubation period of 5–23 days, there may be a vague flu-like illness. The importance of T. *gondii* infection is that, worldwide, it accounts for 70% of cases of chorioretinitis. Immunity halts the progression of infection but the organism is not completely eradicated.

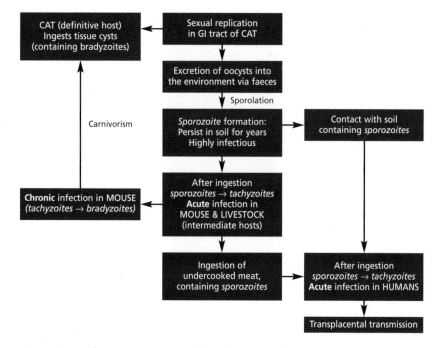

Figure 10.1 Toxoplasmosis gondii replication cycle

Rather, it changes into the slowly replicating bradyzoite, leading to well-demarcated tissue cysts which remain in the host indefinitely and may become reactivated if immunity is subsequently compromised.

Immunity to toxoplasmosis varies worldwide. Seroprevalence is higher in several Latin-American and West African countries compared with Europe and lowest in South West Asia, China and Korea. Seroprevalence has fallen over recent decades: in France from 80–90% to 50–60%, in Sweden from 34% to 18% and in the UK from 22% to 8%. As a result, more women are susceptible to infection during pregnancy.[9]

Vertical transmission of *T. gondii* leads to congenital infection. The placenta acts as a reservoir for the tachyzoites of acute infection and, without maternal treatment, subsequent fetal infection will ensue. It takes between 4 and 8 weeks for infection to pass to the fetus. The risk of fetal infection varies with gestational age. Infection preconception carries a risk of fetal infection of around 1%. Infection in the first, second and third trimesters carry risk of 10–25%, 30–54% and 60–65%, respectively.[10] Indeed, the estimate of risk of fetal infection for pregnant women acquiring infection just before delivery is in the region of 80%. In contrast to the increasing risk of fetal infection with advancing gestational age, the risk of clinical lesions, affecting the brain and eye, declines with increasing gestation. Clinical signs are evident in 60–80% of cases of first-trimester infection compared with 5% in cases of infection acquired before delivery. The most severe outcomes observed following infection in early pregnancy are miscarriage, fetal growth restriction, preterm labour and severe congenital disease. The highest frequency of severe anomalies occurs in children born to mothers who had primary infection between 10 and 24 weeks of gestation.[11]

The most common sequelae of congenital infection are intracranial calcification and chorioretinitis. Ultrasound features of congenital infection include intracerebral calcifications, microcephaly, hydrocephalus and ventricular dilatation. Seventy to ninety percent of congenitally infected newborns are asymptomatic and the classical triad of chorioretinitis, intracerebral calcifications and hydrocephalus is found in less than 10%. Over 95% of children with congenital toxoplasmosis seem to be developmentally normal.

DIAGNOSIS

The following investigations can be employed to diagnose toxoplasmosis: serological testing, PCR, histological demonstration or isolation of the organism. *T. gondii*-specific IgG usually appears 1–2 weeks following infection, peaks within 1–2 months and falls at a variable rate thereafter. IgG antibodies generally persist lifelong. The IgG antibody titre has no correlation with disease severity. The most reliable indicator of maternal toxoplasmosis infection is seroconversion on IgG testing. The traditional test for *T. gondii*-specific IgG is the Sabin-Feldman dye test. However, this can only be performed in reference laboratories with the ability to generate living parasites, since it relies on lysis of the live organisms by the patient's own specific *T. gondii* antibody. This reaction facilitates the uptake of dye into the damaged tissue. Enzyme immunoassays (such as enzyme-linked immunosorbent assay, ELISA) are the most common method used for detection of *T. gondii*-specific IgG.

T. gondii-specific IgM antibodies are detected at an earlier stage, within a few days of infection. They peak at around 1 month and are usually negative within a few months of infection. However, on occasion, IgM antibodies will remain detectable years after the primary infection, which can make differentiation between acute and chronic infection problematic. Persistence of IgM antibodies represents chronic infection and does not appear to have any clinical relevance. IgM, IgA, and IgE antibodies can be measured by the 'double-sandwich' or 'immuno-capture' ELISA method. IgA antibodies follow a similar pattern to IgM antibodies and have little to add in the diagnosis of adult toxoplasmosis infection. Where they are of proven use is in the diagnosis of congenital toxoplasmosis. Immunoglobulin E (IgE) antibodies persist for a shorter period of time in the circulation than IgM and IgA and may be helpful in defining recently acquired infection. IgE is not informative in the assessment of fetal or newborn samples.

The differential agglutination test relies on the differing antigenic properties of acute phase and long-term infection. By comparing the ratio of acute with long-term antigens it may be possible to distinguish acute from chronic infection. In reality, a combination of tests is used to diagnose infection.

As discussed in the section on CMV, avidity testing can be of use when there is uncertainty about the timing of infection. Urea is used to disassociate toxoplasmosis antigen-antibody complexes. The strength of IgG binding increases with the duration of infection. High avidity results suggest infection took place at least 3–5 months earlier. However, low avidity antibodies may persist for many months and so a low avidity result cannot always be assumed to indicate recent infection.

Diagnosis of congenital infection

PCR amplification of amniotic fluid to detect *T. gondii* DNA is the mainstay of diagnosis of congenital infection and, as in the case of CMV infection, has replaced the more invasive technique of fetal blood sampling for this indication. The sensitivity of amniotic fluid PCR for congenital diagnosis is 70–80%, independent of the type of PCR assay used.[12] False negative results do occur. They may be explained by delayed placentitis, delay between placentitis and transmission to the fetus or intermittent presence of the parasite in amniotic fluid. The specificity of PCR is frequently 100% and has not been less than 94%. It is the best available method for prenatal diagnosis.

Recommendations about the timing of amniocentesis in relation to maternal infection vary from immediately to a delay of 4 weeks following diagnosis. Certainly, PCR of amniotic fluid should not be carried out in the absence of serologic, clinical or ultrasound evidence of infection. Amniocentesis is associated with a procedure-related loss risk in the region of 1%. The rationale for proving fetal infection was to be able to change the antibiotic regimen prescribed to the pregnant woman. The fact that there is no evidence that such a change in antibiotic regime is beneficial has to be considered when weighing up the risks of the procedure.

TREATMENT

The aim of drug therapy is two-fold: first, to reduce the risk of vertical transmission to the fetus and, second, if the fetus is infected, to reduce the clinical manifestations of that infection. Spiramycin, a macrolide antibiotic, is used to prevent fetal infection. It concentrates in the placenta and placental drug levels are significantly higher than either maternal or fetal blood levels. The dose is 1 g three times daily and it is commenced upon diagnosis of infection or, alternatively, pending maternal diagnosis so as not to miss the 'window of opportunity' for treatment. Following confirmation of fetal infection by amniotic fluid PCR, therapy can be changed to a combination of the folic acid antagonist, pyrimethamine, and a sulphonamide (such as sulfadiazine) in an attempt to limit fetal damage. One regimen is pyrimethamine in a dose of 50 mg daily and sulfadiazine 3 g daily in divided doses. Folic acid supplementation (leucovorin 10–25 mg daily) is recommended to prevent bone marrow suppression. The pyrimethamine–sulphonamide combination is alternated at 3-weekly intervals with spiramycin for the remainder of pregnancy.

Spiramycin is relatively free from adverse effects and is not teratogenic. Pyrimethamine has been reported to be teratogenic in animal studies but no equivalent studies are available in humans. It might be reasonable to avoid it in the first trimester, when spiramycin can be used as an alternative. The pyrimethamine–sulphonamide combination is associated with a dose-related effect on bone marrow suppression and severe allergic reaction. So treatment is not without potential toxic effects.

It is important to recognise that the efficacy of drug therapy to prevent infection or reduce its sequelae is not established. No randomised controlled trials have been performed to address this issue. Meta-analysis of cohort studies has suggested a weak association between early treatment (within 3 weeks of seroconversion) and reduced risk of congenital toxoplasmosis. There was no evidence that prenatal treatment reduced the risk of clinical manifestations in infected liveborn infants.[13] A randomised controlled clinical trial is the only way to establish whether or not prenatal treatment is of any benefit and there are obviously ethical issues arising from such a proposal.

PRENATAL SCREENING

A number of countries have routine prenatal screening programmes to detect cases of toxoplasmosis infection in pregnancy. These rely on regular testing of women who have been shown to be *T. gondii* seronegative and who are therefore at risk. Frequency of screening varies in different countries from monthly testing (France and Switzerland) to 3-monthly testing (Austria, Germany and Italy). The benefit of monthly testing is that infection will be picked up earlier, allowing swift implementation of drug therapy. However, with the increased number of prenatal visits, more women will have a false-positive result and this number of false-positive results will be greater in those countries with the lowest incidence of maternal infection.

Screening has not been implemented in the UK. The incidence of congenital toxoplasmosis in the UK is approximately 1/10 000 live births with

> **BOX 10.1 PREVENTION OF TOXOPLASMOSIS: ADVICE FOR PREGNANT WOMEN**
>
> - Wear gloves for changing cat litter and gardening, if these activities cannot be avoided, and pay attention to thorough hand hygiene.
> - Do not handle stray cats.
> - Wash hands after handling raw meat.
> - Do not eat undercooked or cured meats.
> - Wash all fruit, vegetables and salads.
> - Do not drink unpasteurised milk or eat unpasteurised milk products.
> - Avoid lambing ewes, newborn lambs and their placentas.

a rate of severe neurological impairment in infancy of less than 5%. In contrast, the incidence of congenital toxoplasmosis in France is 10/10 000 live births. There are several factors to be considered in the decision not to implement screening:[9,14]

- The cost of a screening programme depends on the number of women eligible for testing. In France, where 54% of women are immune, the number of women requiring serial testing is obviously significantly fewer than would be the case in the UK, where only 10% of women are immune to *T. gondii*.
- As discussed above, testing is associated with a false-positive rate.
- Predicting the timing of infection can be difficult: many women will have been infected before conception, when there is minimal risk of congenital infection.
- There is a lack of evidence for a latent phase, when treatment might prevent transmission of the parasite or fetal organ damage.
- At present, there is no treatment of proven benefit in the reduction of vertical transmission or clinical complications.

Primary prevention is an important strategy for limiting the morbidity and mortality associated with toxoplasmosis infection. The extent to which health care strategies are effective remains to be clarified. Current advice for pregnant women is detailed in Box 10.1.

HIV

Globally, in 2008, there were 33.4 million people living with HIV.[15,16] At least 40% of this figure is represented by women of childbearing age. In 2008, there were an estimated 83,000 people in the UK living with HIV (both diagnosed and undiagnosed), contributing to a cumulative total of 108,766 cases reported by the end of 2009.[16] Around 27% of people with HIV are unaware of their diagnosis.[17,18] Since the mid-1990s, the contribution that heterosexual transmission has made to HIV figures has increased significantly.

In 2009, 743 children were born to women who were HIV positive. This is in contrast to 124 children in 1994 and 257 children in 1999.[17] However, the proportion of babies infected with HIV has fallen dramatically, reflecting the impact of antiretroviral therapy. In areas covered by unlinked anonymous screening, 2.1/1000 women giving birth in 2008 (0.21%) were HIV positive.[18] This equates to approximately one in every 486 women giving birth.[18] London continues to have the highest prevalence of pregnancies in HIV positive women (0.37%) but this has been stable since 2004.[18] The prevalence of HIV among women giving birth in the rest of England has increased five-fold since the year 2000.[18] The prevalence of HIV is highest in women born in sub-Saharan Africa, Central America and the Caribbean. Routine antenatal screening, introduced throughout the UK and Ireland from 1999 onwards, means that more than 90% of women are diagnosed before giving birth.

Vertical transmission can occur in the antepartum, intrapartum and post-partum periods. In Africa, approximately one-third of the cases of vertical transmission occur in the postpartum period, reflecting the impact of breastfeeding. In developed countries, up to 75% of transmission occurs intrapartum, as a result of ascending infection from cervicovaginal secretions and fetal exposure to secretions and blood. Cell-free HIV can be isolated in vaginal secretions in up to 40% of women infected with the virus. *In utero* infection can also result from transplacental passage of the virus and direct spread to the amniotic fluid. HIV-1 has been isolated from amniotic fluid, cord blood, first-trimester products of conception and placenta.

FACTORS AFFECTING VERTICAL TRANSMISSION

There are many factors which affect vertical transmission:[19]

- Maternal immune status: there is a linear correlation between falling maternal CD4 count and increasing risk of vertical transmission.
- Increasing viral load increases the risk, although the threshold RNA level for transmission has not been established.
- New seroconversion during pregnancy or in the postnatal period while breastfeeding increases transmission rates.
- Prenatal diagnostic tests: amniocentesis, chorionic villus sampling and fetal blood sampling are associated with a two-fold increase in vertical transmission. Antiretroviral therapy should be given to cover these procedures.

- Elective caesarean section: caesarean section performed before labour or rupture of the membranes results in a 50–70% reduction in vertical transmission rates.[20,21] However, the protective effect of caesarean section was established before the introduction of combination antiretroviral therapy, which has obviously had its own significant impact on transmission rates (see below).
- Duration of membrane rupture: a greater than 4-hour interval following membrane rupture doubles the risk of vertical transmission. It has been estimated that the transmission rate increases by 2% per hour of ruptured membranes up to 24 hours.[22]
- Drug use: this may be independently associated with an increased risk of transmission.
- Zidovudine antiretroviral therapy: the ACTG076 trial compared zidovudine commenced from the start of the second trimester, given intravenously during labour and to the neonate for the first 6 weeks of life, with placebo. The vertical transmission rate in the treatment arm was 8.3% compared with 25.5% in the placebo group, representing a reduction in transmission rate of approximately two-thirds.[23]
- Highly-active antiretroviral therapy (HAART) has been available for women infected with HIV since 1997. There has been a significant increase in the proportion of women receiving HAART before pregnancy: 5% in 1997, 85% in 2003. As a result, the prevalence of undetectable HIV RNA levels has risen from 29% in 1998 to 50% in 2003. Prepregnancy therapy is associated with higher rates of undetectable HIV RNA compared with therapy commenced during pregnancy.[24] The rate of mother-to-child transmission for women on HAART is 1.2% compared with 11.5% for untreated mothers. The risk of transmission is 0.25% if treatment is started before pregnancy and 1.92% when treatment is started during pregnancy. For women on HAART, maternal viral load continues to be the dominant risk factor for vertical transmission, with an odds ratio for transmission of 12.1 (95% CI 2.51–58.6) for viral loads greater than 1000 copies/ml. Elective caesarean section reduces the risk of transmission by two-thirds (OR 0.33, 95% CI 0.11–0.94). In this study, elective caesarean section also reduced the risk of transmission in those women with undetectable HIV RNA (OR 0.07, 95% CI 0.02–0.31) but the small numbers precluded any definitive comment regarding the effect of mode of delivery for those women in this group taking HAART.

There is no clear evidence that any of the following affect vertical transmission rates: race, age, presence of sexually transmitted diseases, the presence of maternal HIV-specific antibodies, episiotomy or fetal scalp electrodes.

TREATMENT IN PREGNANCY

Antiretroviral therapy

The British HIV Association has produced guidelines for the use of anti-retroviral therapy during pregnancy.[25] Women requiring antiretroviral therapy on the grounds of their own health or clinical symptoms should be prescribed HAART, a combination of three or more antiretroviral agents, commencing after the first trimester. Women who have been taking HAART before conception should continue it throughout pregnancy.

Women with low-level viraemia (less than 10 000 HIV RNA copies/ml), a CD4 count of 200–350 cells/microlitre and who wish to be delivered by elective caesarean section can be offered zidovudine monotherapy from 28 weeks of gestation. An alternative regimen is short-term triple anti-retroviral therapy, again commencing from mid-pregnancy. Both therapies are discontinued following delivery, ideally with a viral load of less than 50 copies/ml. HAART should be given to women with a baseline viraemia of greater than 10 000 HIV RNA copies/ml from 28 weeks of gestation. HAART should also be given to women as an alternative to zidovudine and elective caesarean section.

Drug considerations

Nevirapine, a non-nucleoside reverse transcriptase inhibitor is associated with high rates of resistance after single-dose exposure and it is not recommended for use in pregnancy in women with a CD4 count greater than 250 cells/microlitre. The high rates of resistance are attributable to its long half-life. This needs to be borne in mind when discontinuing combination therapy that includes nevirapine. If all drugs are stopped simultaneously, there will be a prolonged exposure to nevirapine, in effect as a single agent, owing to its longer clearance time from the circulation. This increases the risk of subsequent resistance. In addition, nevirapine can be associated with severe hepatotoxicity. A protease inhibitor can be used as an alternative to nevirapine as part of combination therapy. There has been some concern about a link with glucose intolerance but this is not conclusive. HAART has been associated with an increased risk of preterm delivery, compared with no treatment (OR 2.6, 95% CI 1.43–4.75).[26]

Obstetric issues

Elective caesarean section should be offered to women on zidovudine monotherapy and to women on combined therapy with detectable viral load (more than 50 copies/ml).[25] Elective caesarean section should be offered to women co-infected with hepatitis C. Delivery should take place between 38 and 39 weeks of gestation. As discussed above, the beneficial effects of elective caesarean section for women with a viral load of less than 50 copies/ml are unclear and the risks of operative delivery have to be balanced against the potential for no benefit in reducing vertical transmission. Elective vaginal delivery is an option for women on HAART with no detectable viraemia. Obstetric interventions such as amniotomy and fetal scalp electrodes should be avoided. Delivery should be expedited if there is prelabour rupture of the membranes, obviously with some consideration of gestational age.

Syphilis

While syphilis is rarely encountered during pregnancy, there is evidence of a 19-fold increase in the number of cases of syphilis diagnosed at genitourinary medicine clinics between 1998 and 2007.[27] A significant proportion of cases were in women and heterosexual men.

Syphilis results from infection by the spirochaete *Treponema pallidum* during sexual contact. Clinical manifestations are described in a number of stages (Table 10.1). The initial incubation period is 10–90 days. Pregnancy does not alter the clinical course of syphilis. However, syphilis infection can have a seriously adverse impact on pregnancy as will be discussed below.

Vertical transmission can occur via the transplacental route and by contact with genital lesions present in the birth canal. Breastfeeding is not a risk factor for transmission unless there is an infected lesion present on the breast. Spirochaetes have been identified in fetal tissue from as early as 9–10 weeks of gestation and in amniotic fluid from 14 weeks of preg-

Table 10.1 Clinical features of syphilis infection

Type	Time after exposure	Stage
Early (infectious)	9–90 days	Primary
	6 weeks – 6 months (4–8 weeks after primary lesion)	Secondary
	≤ 2 years	Early latent
Late (non-infectious)	> 2 years	Late latent
	3–20 years	Tertiary, gummatous, cardiovascular, neurosyphilis
Congenital	< 2 years since birth	Early congenital (rhinitis, periostitis, mucous patches, hepatosplenomegaly, lymphadenopathy, thrombocytopenia, ocular involvement)
	≥ 2 years since birth	Late congenital (frontal bossing, Clutton joints, interstitial keratitis, teeth deformities, deafness, gummatous involvement)

nancy. If maternal syphilis remains untreated, there is a risk of spontaneous miscarriage, fetal growth restriction, non-immune hydrops fetalis, fetal death, premature delivery and neonatal death. In addition, congenital infection in surviving children is associated with serious sequelae.[28,29]

The risk of congenital infection is related to the stage of maternal infection and is highest in early compared with late disease. Early untreated syphilis of less than 4 years' duration was associated with rates of congenital syphilis, stillbirth and neonatal death of 41%, 25% and 14%, respectively. In this group, 18% of babies were healthy term infants. In contrast, women with latent syphilis had rates of congenital infection, stillbirth and neonatal death of 2%, 12% and 9%, respectively, with 77% of babies healthy at term.[30] In another study, women with late latent syphilis had stillbirth and congenital infection rates each of 10%, compared with rates of 50% for each complication in women with primary or secondary disease.[31]

MATERNAL DIAGNOSIS

The immune response to syphilis involves production of both non-specific antibodies (cardiolipin or lipoidal antibodies) and specific anti-treponemal antibodies. Specific anti-treponemal IgM is detected approximately 2 weeks post-infection and IgG is present by about 4 weeks. At the onset of symptoms, most patients have detectable anti-treponemal IgG and IgM. Serological tests for syphilis can be divided into non-treponemal and treponemal tests:[32]

Non-treponemal
Venereal Diseases Research Laboratory (VDRL) and rapid plasma regain (RPR) tests detect non-specific treponemal antibody and have sensitivities of 70–80% for primary syphilis and close to 100% for secondary syphilis. They become reactive about 4–8 weeks after infection is acquired and up to 1 week after appearance of a chancre. False-positive results do occur and are more frequent in certain groups of patients: those with systemic lupus erythematosus, pregnancy, malignancy, viral and protozoal infection.

Treponemal
T. pallidum haemagglutination test (TPHA), fluorescent treponemal antibody-absorbed test (FTA-abs) and most enzyme immunoassay tests detect specific treponemal antibody. Enzyme immunoassays have greater than 98% sensitivity and greater than 99% specificity.

The diagnosis of syphilis relies on a screening test to detect treponemal antibody, followed by confirmation of this reactive screening test by additional tests. In the UK, VDRL and TPHA testing in combination has been the standard practice for screening. These tests are being replaced increasingly by enzyme immunoassays that detect treponemal IgG or IgG and IgM. IgG enzyme immunoassays give at least comparable results to the VDRL/TPHA combination. The FTA-abs has been considered the gold standard confirmatory test for syphilis but it is subjective and difficult to standardise. Thus, TPHA and enzyme immunoassays can be used as confirmatory tests, provided that they were not used for the original screening test. Other diagnostic techniques include immunoblotting, PCR and dark-field microscopy.

FETAL DIAGNOSIS

It is highly likely that the fetus will be infected when there is active maternal syphilitic infection. The management plan for therapy is not altered by the presence or absence of fetal infection; rather, it is given in the maternal interest with the added benefit of reducing transplacental transmission. Spirochaetes can be detected in amniotic fluid using PCR and fetal blood sampling may show evidence of anaemia, thrombocytopenia and deranged liver function tests. However, invasive testing will not affect the decision to implement therapy and so it is not justified. There are various ultrasound parameters suggestive of fetal infection. These include hydrops, polyhydramnios, placentomegaly, hepatosplenomegaly and non-continuous gastrointestinal obstruction.

TREATMENT

A single dose of benzathine benzylpenicillin (penicillin G) 2.4 million units (1.8 g) is effective in most cases. Failures have been reported in early-stage maternal disease, cases with high RPR/VDRL titres and third-trimester treatment. If treatment is initiated in the third trimester, a second dose of benzathine benzylpenicillin is recommended 1 week later. There is limited information about the efficacy of treatments which are not penicillin-based: ceftriaxone, azithromycin and erythromycin.

Additional treatment will be required for the neonate whose mother was treated less than 4 weeks before delivery, where inadequate antenatal treatment is suspected (for example, commencing in the third trimester) and where non-penicillin therapy was used.[33]

Rubella

The association between first-trimester maternal rubella infection and the congenital rubella syndrome was described by the Australian ophthalmologist Norman Gregg in 1941.[34] He reported congenital cataracts in 78 infants born to mothers who had contracted rubella infection in early pregnancy. Rubella is the first established viral teratogen and the impact of this virus is significant. Rubella caused more birth defects in one year following an outbreak in the USA than thalidomide did during its entire marketing history.[35]

Rubella is an RNA togavirus, first isolated in tissue culture in 1962. It is spread via the respiratory system and has an incubation period of 14–21 days. It is infectious from 7 days before to 10 days after the rash appears. The clinical features are general malaise, lymphadenopathy, a fine generalised macular rash and arthritis. The infection generally runs a benign course.

The serious consequences of rubella infection are encountered when the infection is contracted during early pregnancy. Maternal viraemia occurs 5–7 days after contact and it is during this phase that transplacental infection via haematogenous spread may occur. Viraemia is a prerequisite for congenital infection. Viraemia starts 6–7 days before onset of the rash and ends 1–2 days following its appearance. There are three characteristic features of congenital rubella: congenital heart disease, cataracts and deafness. Ventricular septal defects, patent ductus arteriosus, pulmonary stenosis and coarctation of the aorta are the typical heart defects described. In addition to this triad, fetal growth restriction, mental restriction, microcephaly and neurological abnormalities are recognised consequences of rubella infection during pregnancy.[36] The most important factor influencing the risk of congenital rubella syndrome is the gestational age at which the infection is acquired (Table 10.2).[37] Viraemia in the first trimester is associated with the greatest risk of congenital rubella.

The risk falls substantially if infection is acquired in the second trimester and there are no documented cases of congenital rubella following infection after 20 weeks of gestation. Similarly, infection before the estimated date of conception is without risk.[38,39] The type of anomaly is also influenced by the gestational age at infection. Cataracts occur with infection between 3 and 8 weeks of gestation, cardiac defects between

Table 10.2 Rates of intrauterine transmission and risk of adverse fetal outcome for rubella infection in pregnancy (adapted from Morgan-Capner et al. 2002)[37]

Gestational age	Risk of intrauterine transmission (%)	Risk of adverse fetal outcome (%)
< 11 weeks	90	90
11–16 weeks	55	20
16–20 weeks	45	Minimal
> 20 weeks	45	No increased risk

3 and 10 weeks of gestation and infection from 16–20 weeks of gestation is likely to be associated with deafness only.[40–42] The rate of low-birthweight babies (less than 10th centile) is significantly higher in seropositive compared with seronegative infants and this effect is most dramatic when rubella is contracted in the first trimester.[38]

The National Congenital Rubella Surveillance Programme records all cases of congenital rubella in the UK. Before the introduction of rubella vaccination in 1970, there were approximately 200–300 congenital rubella births in non-epidemic years, with significantly more cases in epidemic years. Following the introduction of vaccination in 1970, the number of congenital rubella births has fallen from approximately 50/year (1971–75) to an average of 20/year (1986–90). Between 1991 and 2002, there have been only 40 reported cases of congenital rubella.[43]

The evolution of vaccination programmes in the UK is illustrated in Box 10.2. As a result of such programmes, the rate of congenital rubella in the developed world has become vanishingly small. However, the mothers of the very few cases that continue to occur seem to fall into three categories:

- those who acquired infection abroad in early pregnancy (Africa and Asia for the majority)
- those born abroad but acquired infection in the UK, often within 2 years of arrival
- UK-born women, a proportion of whom have not been previously immunised.

Maintaining a low level and therefore a low risk of infection relies upon a high level of immunity in the population as a whole. It is important to consider the following:[43]

- The uptake of MMR vaccination, the most effective way to control all three diseases, has fallen by over 10% since 1995.
- Single rubella vaccination is no longer available.
- Outbreaks of rubella infection abroad can result in outbreaks in the UK.

BOX 10.2   RUBELLA VACCINATION PROGRAMMES

1970   Rubella vaccine offered to schoolgirls in the UK

1970s Antenatal screening and postpartum vaccination of susceptible women

1988   Measles, mumps and rubella (MMR) vaccination introduced for all infants at 12–15 months of age

1996   Schoolgirl vaccination discontinued
       Second dose of MMR for preschool children introduced

- Women from ethnic minorities in the UK have higher susceptibility to infection than white women in the UK and this may be compounded by low vaccine uptake.

There is therefore a need to maintain vigilance about rubella screening and vaccination of susceptible women if the low rates of congenital infection, a potentially preventable condition, are to be sustained. There are no cases of fetal damage following inadvertent vaccination during pregnancy.

DIAGNOSIS

At least 50% of cases of rubella are asymptomatic and clinical diagnosis is unreliable owing to the mild and non-specific features of the illness. Accurate diagnosis depends upon laboratory investigations. The diagnosis is established by serological testing, most commonly using ELISA. In acute infection, rubella-specific IgM appears about 5 days after the rash and usually persists for 6 weeks. Rubella-specific IgG is generally detected 2–3 weeks after the onset of infection. Occasionally, IgM can persist in the circulation for a year or more following natural infection, reactivation of infection or vaccination. For this reason, a positive IgM in isolation should not be interpreted as an acute infection without the addition of further investigations. Acute infection can be confirmed by a significant rise in IgG on paired samples, virus isolation or IgG avidity testing. The presence of rubella-specific IgG antibodies with high avidity rules out a recent infection. It is estimated that results from about 2% of serum samples tested for rubella IgM will be difficult to interpret.[44] In addition, false-positive IgM results can occur in association with parvovirus infection, mononucleosis and rheumatoid factor. The control of rubella infection in the UK means that most rubella-specific IgM results do not reflect acute infection.

Rubella reinfection, although rare, is a recognised entity and refers to reinfection in a person who has had a previous documented primary infection or successful immunisation. Most cases of reinfection are asymptomatic and viraemia is rare. The risk of congenital damage in the fetus following reinfection during the first 16 weeks of pregnancy is undetermined but is likely to be low.[45]

FETAL DIAGNOSIS

Since maternal infection in the first trimester is associated with such a high rate of fetal abnormality, it is likely that termination of pregnancy will be the chosen management option: there is no treatment for congenital rubella. However, the risk of fetal damage is much less with infection between 13 and 16 weeks of gestation and it is in this situation that information about fetal infection is invaluable for decision-making purposes. As in the case of CMV infection, it is important to perform the diagnostic tests at the correct time interval from maternal infection. Fetal sampling of either amniotic fluid (reverse transcriptase PCR) or fetal blood (serology or RNA) should not be performed until 6–8 weeks following maternal infection. Fetal production of IgM cannot be relied upon before 22 weeks of gestation and renal excretion of the virus is not established until about 21 weeks of gestation. These factors have to be borne in mind if false-negative results are to be avoided. The procedure-related risks have to be balanced against the low risk of fetal damage when infection occurs after mid-gestation.

Varicella zoster

Varicella zoster (VZV), a DNA virus, is a member of the herpes family of viruses. Primary infection with the virus causes chickenpox. Following this primary infection the virus remains latent, residing in dorsal root ganglion cells, and reactivation results in herpes zoster (shingles). Varicella zoster is highly contagious and has an incubation period of 14–21 days. The illness comprises fever, general malaise and a characteristic maculopapular rash. The infectious period is from 48 hours before onset of the rash until the vesicles have crusted over. At least 90% of adults in the UK are immune (VZV IgG positive).

Varicella infection during pregnancy is uncommon (1/2000 pregnancies) but can have implications for the fetus or neonate. The following discussion focuses on fetal varicella syndrome (FVS). There is a risk of FVS if maternal chickenpox and viraemia occur in the first 20 weeks of pregnancy. The syndrome was first described in 1947 and results from the reactivation of the virus *in utero*. FVS is the result of herpes zoster and not the primary infection. There is, therefore, a very short latency between primary infection and reactivation, thought to be due to the immaturity of the fetal immune system. This theory of reactivation is supported by the fact that FVS is characterised by skin lesions in a dermatomal distribution, as is the case in adult shingles. FVS can only occur following primary maternal infection. Localised herpes zoster in pregnancy does not cause fetal or neonatal infection. It is uncertain whether disseminated zoster in the immunocompromised mother carries a fetal or neonatal risk. The risk of fetal varicella syndrome following maternal chickenpox is gestation dependent: 0.4% if infection occurs less than 12 weeks and 2% if infection occurs between 13 and 20 weeks of gestation. There is no risk of FVS if infection occurs after 20 weeks of pregnancy.[46] Infection after 20 weeks of gestation can lead to fetal infection but it does not cause FVS. Fetal infection in the second half of pregnancy may first become apparent as herpes zoster in infancy or early childhood, following reactivation of the virus. First-trimester varicella infection does not increase the risk of miscarriage.

Fetal varicella syndrome has a neonatal mortality of 30%. Clinical features of the syndrome are skin-scarring in a dermatomal distribution (72%) with associated bone and muscle hypoplasia; neurological defects (62%) and mental restriction; eye diseases (52%): cataracts, microphthalmia and chorioretinitis; gastrointestinal (20%) and genitourinary anomalies (12%).[47] Ultrasound features of FVS include microcephaly, limb hypoplasia and fetal growth restriction (present in 23%). Varicella infection before 20 weeks of gestation is not an indication in itself for termination of pregnancy. Ultrasound and magnetic resonance imaging can be used to identify evidence of these anomalies but there must be an interval of approximately 6 weeks between infection and examination to allow time for these features to develop. Amniotic fluid PCR can detect the virus but a positive result indicates an infected but not necessarily affected fetus. As the risk of FVS is 2% or lower, other features such as ultrasound are essential to detect those infected fetuses that develop FVS.

Varicella zoster immunoglobulin G (VZ IgG) is given to non-immune pregnant women who have had a significant contact (face-to-face for 5 minutes, same room for 15 minutes, contact in a large open ward) during the infectious time period. If immunity is not known, maternal serology can be checked rapidly by the virus laboratory. A person is immune if antibodies are detected in the blood within 10 days of contact. If indicated, VZ IgG is given as soon as possible following contact up to an interval of 10 days. VZ IgG is not given to women who have developed chickenpox. The aim is to reduce the risk of maternal viraemia, fetal infection and fetal varicella syndrome, although it is not wholly preventive.

Parvovirus

Parvovirus infection during pregnancy can cause fetal anaemia, hydrops and fetal death. A number of authors comprehensively review parvovirus and its complications.[48,49] Outbreaks occur every 3–4 years, most commonly in late winter and spring. B19 is the only member of the parvovirus family to be pathogenic in humans. It was identified coincidentally in 1974 when assessing tests for the hepatitis B antigen. It binds to the blood group P-antigen cellular receptor that is present on haematopoietic precursors, endothelial cells, fetal myocytes and placental trophoblast. Its action on the haematopoietic system results in profound anaemia and non-immune hydrops fetalis (NIHF). In addition, viral particles have been identified in fetal myocardial tissue; cardiac dysfunction owing to myocarditis may also contribute to the development of cardiac failure. Approximately 50% of pregnant women are susceptible to infection. Infection in adults is frequently asymptomatic. Infection in children can produce the characteristic 'slapped cheek' appearance

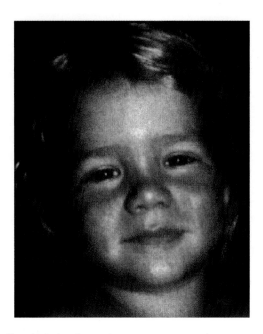

Figure 10.2 Slapped cheek syndrome

illustrated in Figure 10.2. The rate of transplacental transmission is around 30%. The peak incidence of hydrops occurs with infection between 17 and 24 weeks of gestation.[50] Quoted risks for hydrops developing if infection occurs at 9–20 weeks or 13–20 weeks of gestation are 2.9%[51] and 7.1%,[50] respectively. The virus infects the fetal liver, which in the second trimester is the main source of haematopoietic activity. Haematopoiesis is augmented at this gestation to meet the demands of the growing fetus and the lifespan of red blood cells is shorter, rendering the fetus particularly susceptible to any arrest in haematopoiesis. Levels of the P-antigen are negligible in the third trimester so the risk of anaemia and hydrops appears to be low. Fetal infection at any gestation can be asymptomatic. The mean interval from maternal infection to development of NIHF is 2–6 weeks,[52] although longer intervals have been reported.[51]

Parvovirus is responsible for 15–20% of cases of NIHF. The early ultrasound features of hydrops are ascites and cardiomegaly (Figure 10.3). This is followed by skin oedema, pericardial effusions and placental oedema. If there is evidence of progressive hydrops, there is a significant risk of fetal death.

Maternal serology will confirm recent infection. B19-specific IgM peaks at 10–14 days post-infection, declining thereafter over 2–3 months. B19-specific IgG plateaus 4 weeks post-infection. If IgM titres exceed IgG, the

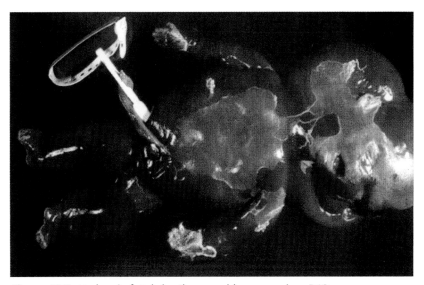

Figure 10.3 Hydropic fetal death caused by parvovirus B19

infection took place within the previous month and the fetus remains at risk of complications, even if none are present at initial presentation.[53] Maternal serology can be misleading if checked earlier than 7 days post-contact, as IgG and IgM could both be negative at this stage. Similarly, by the time of clinically established hydrops, IgM levels may already be low or, rarely, undetectable.[48] PCR techniques for viral DNA are required for diagnosis of fetal infection, rather than fetal serology, but in reality ultrasound is the mainstay of fetal surveillance and diagnosis.

Middle cerebral artery Doppler for the prediction of fetal anaemia is discussed in Chapter 5. This technique is also reliable for the prediction of fetal anaemia secondary to parvovirus infection; sensitivities of 94–100% and specificities of 93–100% have been reported.[54,55] The anaemia can be successfully treated by intrauterine transfusion, which reduces the mortality rate of severe hydrops.[51,56,57] Generally, a single transfusion is required. Cordocentesis and intrauterine transfusion is obviously not without risk and, as for cases of immune anaemia, the risks are higher when the fetus is hydropic. Thrombocytopenia is often a feature of parvovirus infection, which will potentially increase the procedure-related risk of exsanguination. In addition to red cell transfusion, consideration should be given to transfusion of platelets in those fetuses with severe thrombocytopenia.

Close fetal surveillance is required following maternal seroconversion before 24 weeks of gestation. Weekly middle cerebral artery peak systolic velocity measurement should be carried out and intrauterine transfusion

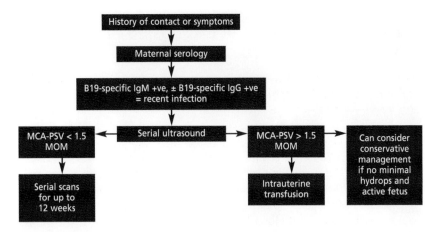

Figure 10.4 Management of parvovirus infection in pregnancy

considered for results above the 1.5 MOM cut-off point. Serial surveillance for 8–12 weeks post-conversion is indicated. Anaemia secondary to parvovirus does have the potential to resolve, as the fetus mounts its own immune response. As a result, middle cerebral artery Doppler monitoring may identify some fetuses that are anaemic at presentation but who are actually in the recovery phase of the infection. If other signs of fetal wellbeing are present, such as good fetal movements and normal liquor volume, it may be possible to continue conservative management and avoid intrauterine transfusion, with its attendant risks, in these particular cases. A proposed management plan is summarised in Figure 10.4.

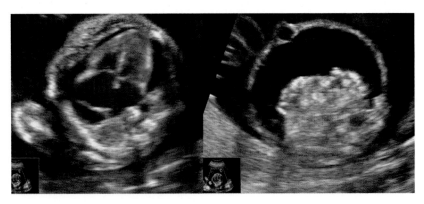

Figure 10.5 Fetal pericardial effusion and ascites secondary to parvovirus B19 infection

The role of ultrasound in diagnosing fetal infection

There are a number of ultrasound features indicative of potential or actual fetal infection. As discussed, specific structural malformations can result from certain viral infections. Non-specific features of congenital infection include fetal growth restriction and NIHF (Figure 10.5). Fetal growth restriction occurs secondary to capillary endothelial damage during organogenesis. Depending on the timing of maternal infection, severe growth restriction may present in the early second trimester. There is often placental damage, which is reflected in abnormal Doppler velocimetry. Chronic hypoxia resulting from uteroplacental dysfunction leads to redistribution of blood flow to vital structures, evidenced by a fall in resistance in the middle cerebral circulation. Continuing deterioration in the fetal condition will lead to abnormal venous waveforms.

A number of congenital infections are complicated by NIHF. Underlying mechanisms for this include fetal anaemia, increased microvascular hydro-static pressure, myocarditis and cardiac dysfunction. Some of the observed features are generalised skin oedema, ascites, pleural and pericardial effusions and placental and umbilical cord oedema. Table 10.3 summarises some of the ultrasound features associated with different viral infections.

Summary

The management of suspected or actual fetal infection can be challenging and is often associated with a number of clinical uncertainties. Table 10.4 summarises information relating to transmission and risk of adverse outcome for the infections that have been discussed. Pitfalls in diagnosis must be recognised and the limitations in predicting long-term outcomes acknowledged. It is important that potentially preventable infections such as rubella are kept under stringent control with vaccination programmes. Screening and preventive treatment for HIV infection has dramatically reduced the risks to the fetus and neonate and this achievement must be sustained. In the case of parvovirus infection, where *in utero* therapy is of proven benefit, maintaining public awareness is essential.

Table 10.3 Ultrasound features of congenital infection

Ultrasound feature	Virus
Intracranial calcification	Cytomegalovirus, toxoplasmosis
Hydrocephalus	Cytomegalovirus, toxoplasmosis
Microcephaly	Cytomegalovirus
Cataracts, chorioretinitis	Rubella, cytomegalovirus, herpes simplex virus, toxoplasmosis
Cardiac: pulmonary stenosis, ventricular septal defect	Rubella
Hepatosplenomegaly	Cytomegalovirus, parvovirus B19, toxoplasmosis, *Treponema pallidum*
Echogenic bowel	Cytomegalovirus, herpes simplex virus, varicella zoster virus, parvovirus B19
Limb defects	Varicella zoster virus, rubella
Fetal growth restriction	Cytomegalovirus, rubella, varicella zoster virus, *T. pallidum*
Non-immune hydrops fetalis	Parvovirus B19, cytomegalovirus, toxoplasmosis, rubella

Table 10.4 Transmission and risk of adverse outcome according to gestation

Infection	Peak transmission	Peak impact
Cytomegalovirus	Not influenced by gestational age	First half of pregnancy
Toxoplasmosis	Third trimester (60–65% risk of transmission)	First trimester (60–80% risk of clinical signs)
HIV	Intrapartum in the developed world	
Syphilis	Risk of congenital infection related to stage of maternal disease, not gestational age	
Rubella	First trimester (90% risk of transmission)	First trimester (90% risk of adverse outcome)
Varicella zoster virus	Not influenced by gestational age	Up to 20 weeks of gestation (2% risk fetal varicella syndrome)
Parvovirus B19	Not influenced by gestational age	9–20 weeks (3% risk of hydrops)

References

1. Ornoy A, Diav-Citrin O. Fetal effects of primary and secondary cytomegalovirus infection in pregnancy. *Reprod Toxicol* 2006;21:399–409.

2. Burny W, Liesnard C, Donner C, Marchant A. Epidemiology, pathogenesis and prevention of congenital cytomegalovirus infection. *Expert Rev Anti Infect Ther* 2004;2:881–94.

3. Revello MG, Gerna G. Diagnosis and management of human cytomegalovirus infection in the mother, fetus, and newborn infant. *Clin Microbiol Rev* 2002;15:680–715.

4. Bodeus M, Hubinont C, Bernard P, Bouckaert A, Thomas K, Goubau P. Prenatal diagnosis of human cytomegalovirus by culture and polymerase chain reaction: 98 pregnancies leading to congenital infection. *Prenat Diagn* 1999;19:314–17.

5. Boppana SB, Pass RF, Britt WJ, Stagno S, Alford CA. Symptomatic congenital cytomegalovirus infection: neonatal morbidity and mortality. *Pediatr Infect Dis J* 1992;11:93–9.

6. Benoist G, Salomon LJ, Jacquemard F, Daffos F, Ville Y. The prognostic value of ultrasound abnormalities and biological parameters in blood of fetuses infected with cytomegalovirus. *BJOG* 2008;115:823–9.

7. Jacquemard F, Yamamoto M, Costa JM, Romand S, Jaqz-Aigrain E, Dejean A, *et al.* Maternal administration of valaciclovir in symptomatic intrauterine cytomegalovirus infection. *BJOG* 2007;114:1113–21.

8. Rorman E, Zamir CS, Rilkis I, Ben-David H. Congenital toxoplasmosis: prenatal aspects of *Toxoplasma gondii* infection. *Reprod Toxicol* 2006;21:458–72.

9. Working Group on Toxoplasma Infection in Pregnancy. Antenatal and newborn screening for toxoplasmosis. Antenatal subcommittee, National Screening Committee 2001 [www.nelh.nhs.uk/screening/antenata_pps/toxoplasmosis.html].

10. Lynfield R, Guerina NG. Toxoplasmosis. *Pediatr Rev* 1997;18:75–83.

11. Remington JS, Desmonts G. Infectious diseases of the fetus and newborn infant. In: Remington JS, Klein JD, editors. *Toxoplasmosis.* 3rd ed. Philadelphia: WB Saunders; 1990. p. 89–195.

12. Bastion P. Molecular diagnosis of toxoplasmosis. *Trans R Soc Trop Med Hyg* 2002;96 Suppl 1:205–15.

13. SYROCOT Study Group. Effectiveness of prenatal treatment for congenital toxoplasmosis: a meta-analysis of individual patients' data. *Lancet* 2007;369:115–22.

14. Gilbert RE, Peckham CS. Congenital toxoplasmosis in the United Kingdom: to screen or not to screen? *J Med Screen* 2002;9:135–41.

15. Terrence Higgins Trust. Information resources. 2010 [www.tht.org.uk/informationresources/factsandstatistics/worldwide].

16. Health Protection Agency. United Kingdom New HIV Diagnoses to end of December 2009 (national tables no. 2) [www.hpa.org.uk/web/HPAweb&HPA webStandard/HPAweb_C/1252660002826].

17. AVERT. Global HIV/AIDS estimates, end of 2008 [http://www.avert.org/worldstats.htm].

18. Health Protection Agency. *HIV in the United Kingdom: 2009 Report*. London: HPA; 2009 [www.hpa.org.uk/webw/HPAweb&HPAwebStandard/HPAweb_C/1259151891866?p=1249920575999].

19. Groginsky E, Bowdler N, Yankowitz J. Update on vertical HIV transmission. *J Reprod Med* 1998;43:637–46.

20. International Perinatal HIV Group. The mode of delivery and the risk of vertical transmission of human immunodeficiency virus type 1: a meta-analysis of 15 prospective cohort studies. *New Engl J Med* 1999;340:977–87.

21. European Mode of Delivery Collaboration. Elective caesarean section versus vaginal delivery in prevention of vertical HIV-1 transmission: a randomised clinical trial. *Lancet* 1999;353:1035–9.

22. International Perinatal HIV Group. Duration of ruptured membranes and vertical transmission of HIV-1: a meta-analysis from 15 prospective cohort studies. *AIDS* 2001;15:357–68.

23. Connor EM, Sperling RS, Gelber R, Kiselev P, Scott G, O'Sullivan MJ, *et al.* Reduction of maternal–infant transmission of human immunodeficiency virus type 1 with zidovudine treatment: Pediatric AIDS Clinical Trials Group Protocol 076 Study Group. *N Engl J Med* 1994;331:1173–80.

24. European Collaborative Study. Mother-to-child transmission of HIV infection in the era of highly active antiretroviral therapy. *Clin Infect Dis* 2005;40:458–65.

25. De Ruiter A, Mercey D, Anderson J, Chakraborty R, Clayden P, Foster G, *et al.* British HIV Association and children's HIV Association guidelines for the management of HIV in pregnant women. *HIV Med* 2008;9:452–502.

26. European Collaborative Study and the Swiss Mother and Child HIV Cohort Study. Combination antiretroviral therapy and duration of pregnancy. *AIDS* 2000;14:2913–20.

27. AVERT. STD statistics and STDs in the UK [www.avert.org/stdstatisticuk.htm].

28. Sanchez PJ, Wendel GD. Syphilis in pregnancy. *Clin Perinatol* 1997;24:71–90.

29. Genc M, Ledger WJ. Syphilis in pregnancy. *Sex Transm Inf* 2000;76:73–9.

30. Ingraham N. The value of penicillin alone in the treatment of congenital syphilis. *Acta Derm Venerol* 1951;31:60–88.

31. Fiumara N, Fleming W, Dowing *et al.* The incidence of prenatal syphilis at the Boston City Hospital. *N Engl J Med* 1952;247:48–52.

32. Egglestone SI, Turner AJL, for the PHLS Syphilis Serology Working Group. Serological diagnosis of syphilis. *Commun Dis Public Health* 2000;3:158–62.

33. Kingston M, French P, Goh B, Goold P, Higgins S, Sukthankar A, *et al.* UK national guidelines on the management of syphilis. *Int J STD AIDS* 2008;19:729–40.

34. Gregg N. Congenital cataract following German measles in the mother. *Trans Ophthalmol Soc Aust* 1941;3:35–46.

35. Webster WS. Teratogen update: congenital rubella. *Teratology* 1998;58:13–23.

36. De Santis M, Cavaliere AF, Straface G, Caruso A. Rubella infection in pregnancy. *Reprod Toxicol* 2006;21:390–8.

37. Morgan-Capner P, Crowcroft NS. Guidelines on the management of, and exposure to, rash illness in pregnancy (including consideration of relevant antibody screening programmes in pregnancy). *Commun Dis Public Health* 2002;5:59–71.

38. Miller E, Cradock-Watson JE, Pollock TM. Consequences of confirmed maternal rubella at successive stages of pregnancy. *Lancet* 1982;ii:781–4.

39. Enders G, Nickerl-Pacher U, Miller E, Cradock-Watson JE. Outcome of confirmed periconceptional maternal rubella. *Lancet* 1988;i:1445–7.

40. Grillner L, Forsgren M, Barr B, Bottiger M, Danielsson L, De Verdier C. Outcome of rubella during pregnancy with special references to the 17th–24th weeks of gestation. *Scand J Infect Dis* 1983;15:321–5.

41. Ueda K, Nishida Y, Oshima K, Shepard TH. Congenital rubella syndrome: correlation of gestational age at time of maternal rubella with type of defect. *J Pediatr* 1979;94:763–5.

42. Ueda K, Hisanaga S, Nishida Y, Shepard TH. Low birth weight and congenital rubella syndrome: effect of gestational age at time of maternal rubella infection. *Clin Pediatr (Phil)* 1981;20:730–3.

43. Tookey P. Rubella in England, Scotland and Wales. *Eurosurveillance* 2004;9(4).

44. Best JM, O'Shea S, Tipples G, Davies N, Al-Khusaiby SM, Krause A, *et al*. Interpretation of rubella serology in pregnancy-pitfalls and problems. *BMJ* 2002;325:147–8.

45. Morgan-Capner P, Miller E, Vurdien JE, Ramsay ME. Outcome of pregnancy after maternal reinfection with rubella. *CDR (Lond Engl Rev)* 1991;1(6):R57–9.

46. Enders G, Miller E, Cradock-Watson J, Bolley I, Ridehalgh M. Consequences of varicella and herpes zoster in pregnancy: prospective study of 1739 cases. *Lancet* 1994;343:1548–51.

47. Sauerbrei A, Wutzler P. Herpes simplex and varicella-zoster virus infections during pregnancy: current concepts of prevention, diagnosis and therapy. Part 2: Varicella-zoster virus infections. *Med Microbiol Immunol* 2007;196:95–102.

48. De Jong EP, de Haan TR, Kroes AC, Beersma MF, Oepkes D, Walther FJ. Parvovirus B19 infection in pregnancy. *J Clin Virol* 2006;36:1–7.

49. Heegaard ED, Brown KE. Human parvovirus B19. *Clin Microbiol Rev* 2002;15:485–505.

50. Enders M, Weidner A, Zoellner I, Searle K, Enders G. Fetal morbidity and mortality after acute human parvovirus B19 infection in pregnancy: prospective evaluation of 1018 cases. *Prenat Diagn* 2004;24:513–18.

51. Miller E, Fairley CK, Cohen BJ, Seng C. Immediate and long term outcome of human parvovirus B19 infection in pregnancy. *Br J Obstet Gynaecol* 1998;105:174-178.

52. Yaegashi N, Niinuma T, Chisaka H, Watanabe T, Uehara S, Okamura K, *et al*. The incidence of, and factors leading to, parvovirus B19-related hydrops fetalis following maternal infection; report of 10 cases and meta-analysis. *J Infect* 1998;37:28–35.

53. Beersma MF, Claas EC, Sopaheluakan T, Kroes AC. B19 viral loads in relation to VP1 and VP2 antibody responses in diagnostic blood samples. *J Clin Virol* 34:71–5.

54. Cosmi E, Mari G, Delle Chiaie L, Detti L, Akiyama M, Murphy J, et al. Noninvasive diagnosis by doppler ultrasonography of fetal anemia resulting from parvovirus infection. *Am J Obstet Gynecol* 2002;187:1290–3.

55. Delle Chiaie L, Buck G, Grab D, Terinde R. Prediction of fetal anemia with Doppler measurement of the middle cerebral artery peak systolic velocity in pregnancies complicated by maternal blood group alloimmunization or parvovirus B19 infection,. *Ultrasound Obstet Gynecol* 2001;18:232–6.

56. Fairley CK, Smoleniec JS, Caul OE, Miller E. Observational study of effect of intrauterine transfusions on outcome of fetal hydrops after parvovirus B19 infection. *Lancet* 1995;346:1335–7.

57. Rodis JF, Rodner C, Hansen AA, Borgida AF, Deoliveira I, Shulman Rosengren S. Long-term outcome of children following maternal human parvovirus B19 infection. *Obstet Gynecol* 1998;91:125–8.

Index

intracranial haemorrhage 62, 92, 128
intraperitoneal transfusion, rhesus
    disease 84, 85, 89–90
intrauterine death of one twin
    dichorionic twins 159–60
    monochorionic twins 160–1
intrauterine growth retardation *see* fetal
    growth restriction
intrauterine transfusion
    after intrauterine death of one twin
        161
    in fetal alloimmune
        thrombocytopenia 92
    in parvovirus B19 infection 195–6
    in rhesus disease 84, 89–91
intravascular transfusion, rhesus disease
    84, 85, 89–91, 92
ischiopagus 169

Jeune syndrome 120

karyotypic abnormalities *see*
    chromosomal abnormalities
karyotyping
    amniocentesis for 23–4
    chorionic villus sampling for 28
    in congenital heart disease 66
    cordocentesis for 29
    in gastrointestinal anomalies 68, 70
    in non-immune hydrops 119
    in renal tract anomalies 74, 94
    in twin pregnancy 159, 162
kidneys
    anomaly scan 38, 42, 51
    cystic disease 44, 73
Kleihauer test 96, 128

lambda sign 154, 155
laser ablation, placental vascular
    anastomoses 99, 107, 163, 165–6
lemon sign 58, 59
leucovorin 181
Liggins GC 79
Liley AW 79
Liley curve 86–7
limb-reduction defects, after chorionic
    villus sampling 27

limbs, anomaly scan 38, 43
lips, anomaly scan 37, 39
lithium therapy 35
lower urinary tract obstruction (LUTO)
    73, 92–5
    antenatal assessment 94
    fetal therapy 94–5
lung lesions, fetal 102–3
lung-to-head ratio, fetal 101

magnetic resonance imaging (MRI),
    fetal
    cytomegalovirus infection 176
    sacrococcygeal teratoma 104, 105
maternal age, Down syndrome
    screening 2–3, 4
Meckel–Gruber syndrome 58
medical fetal therapy 80–1
metabolic disorders, inherited *see* inborn
    errors of metabolism
microcephaly 49, 128, 175
middle cerebral artery (MCA) Doppler
    studies
    in fetal anaemia 87–9, 195–6
    in fetal growth restriction 142
mid-trimester *see* second trimester
mifepristone 127
mirror syndrome, maternal 102, 121
miscarriage
    Down syndrome pregnancies 11–12
    in twin pregnancy 159–60
    see also fetal loss
misoprostol 126, 127
monoamniotic twins 153, 154, 168
monochorionic twin pregnancy 153
    antenatal determination 154–6
    chorionic villus sampling 30
    complications 107–8, 160–9
    embryology 153–4
    intrauterine death of one twin
        160–1
    management 170
    selective feticide 107–8, 132, 162, 163
    see also chorionicity
mosaicism 23
    confined placental 28, 30
    true fetal 23, 28